Vaccines - the History and Future

Edited by Vijay Kumar

Published in London, United Kingdom

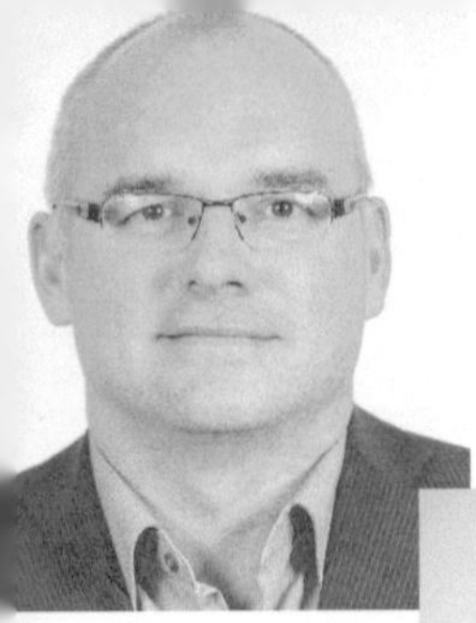

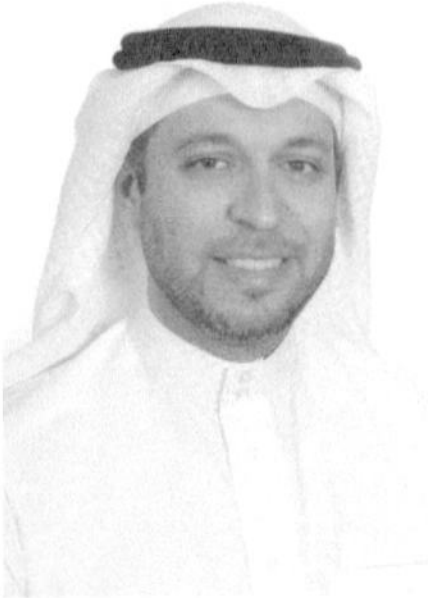

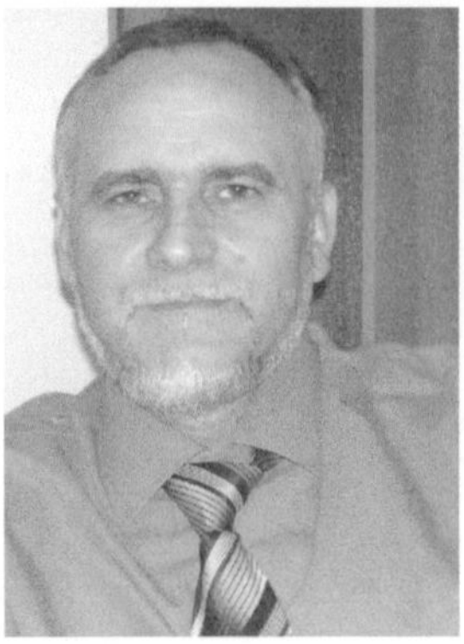

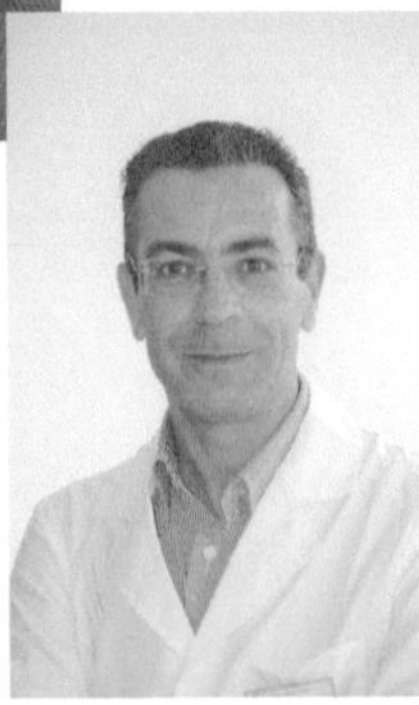

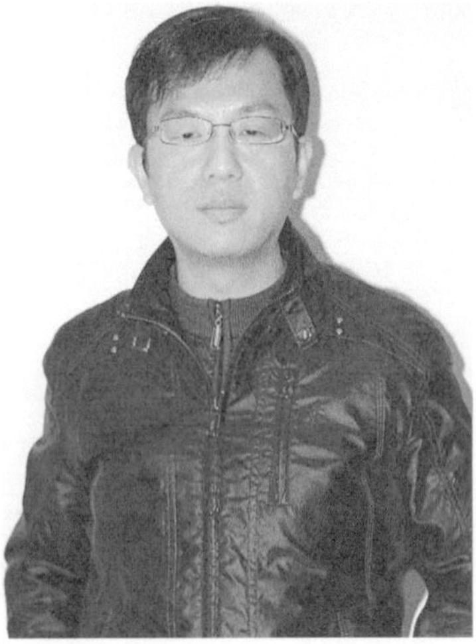

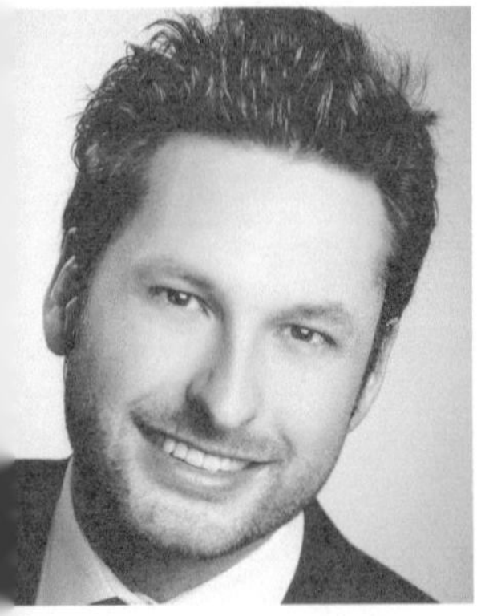

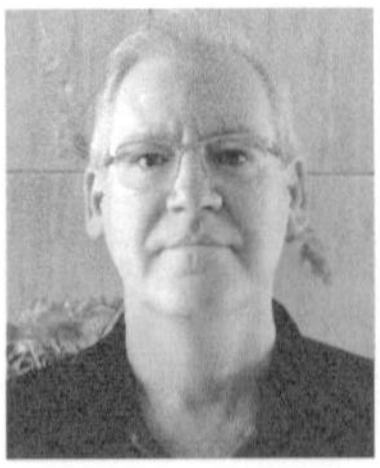

IntechOpen

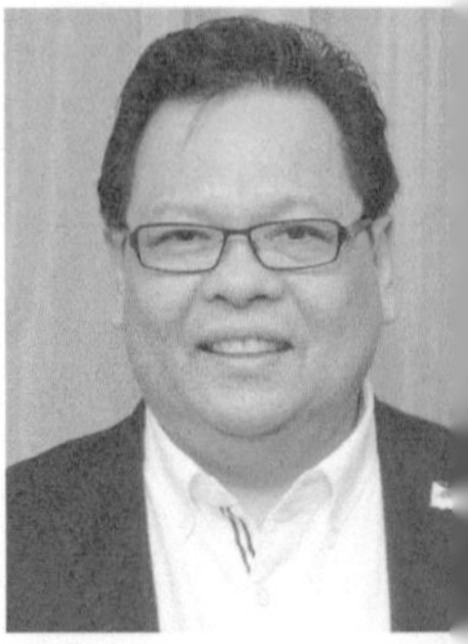

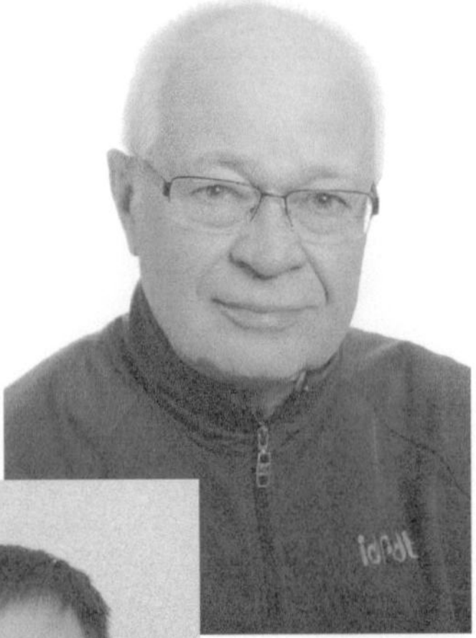

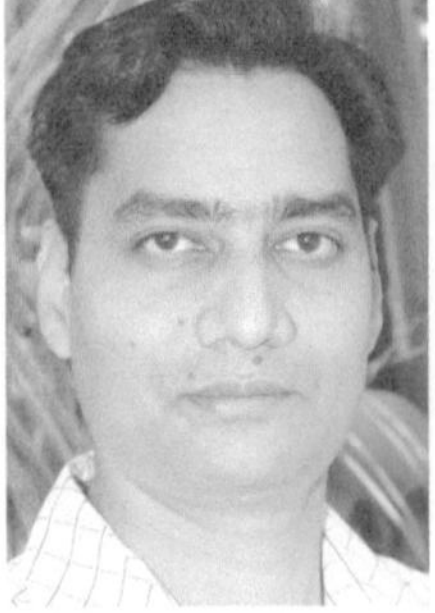

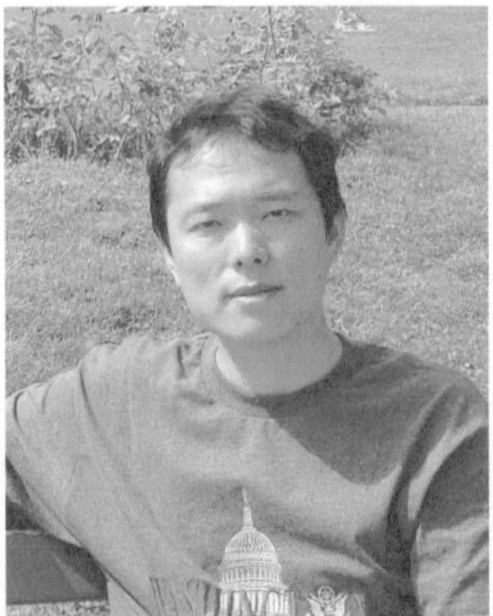

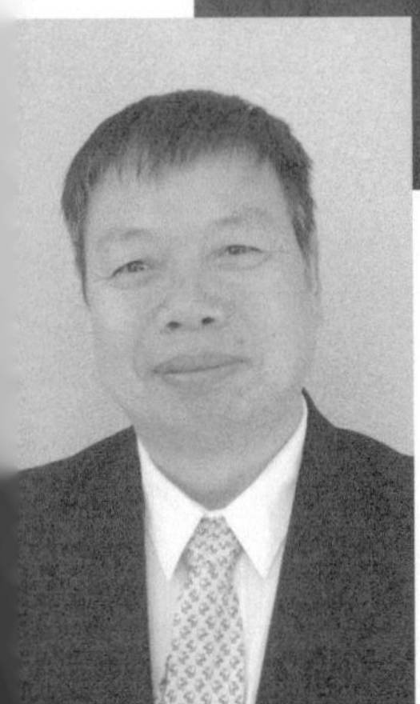

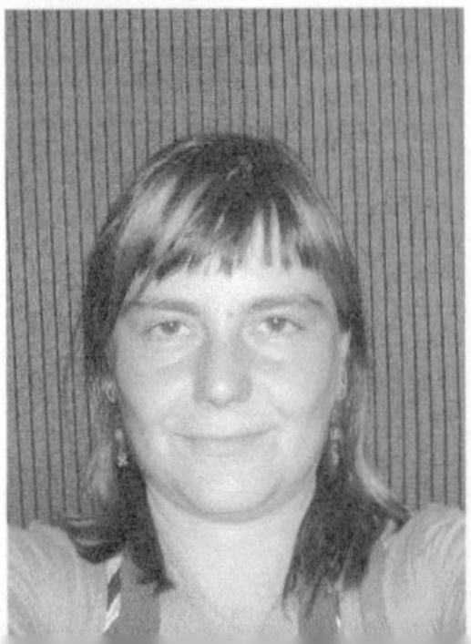

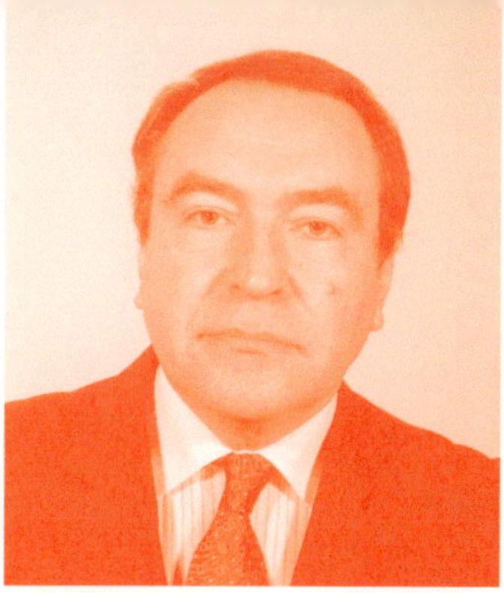
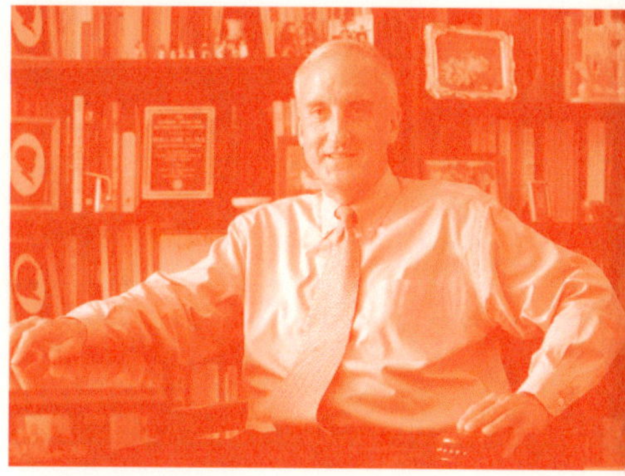
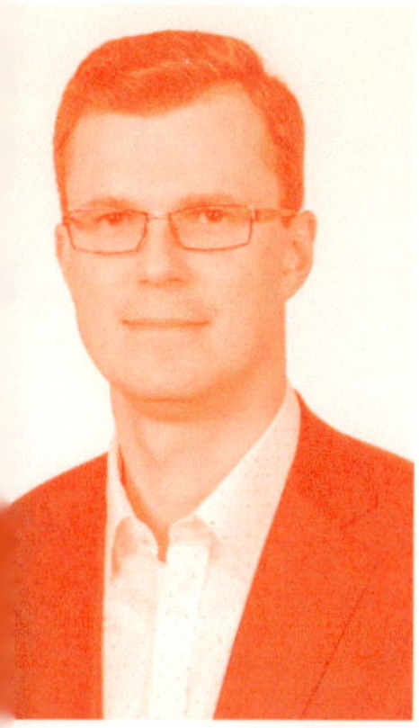
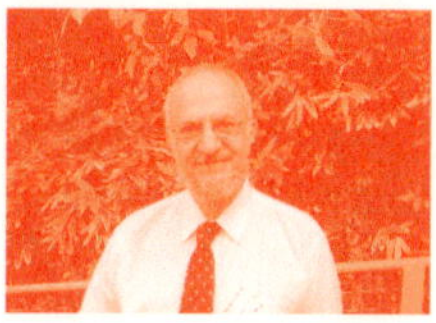
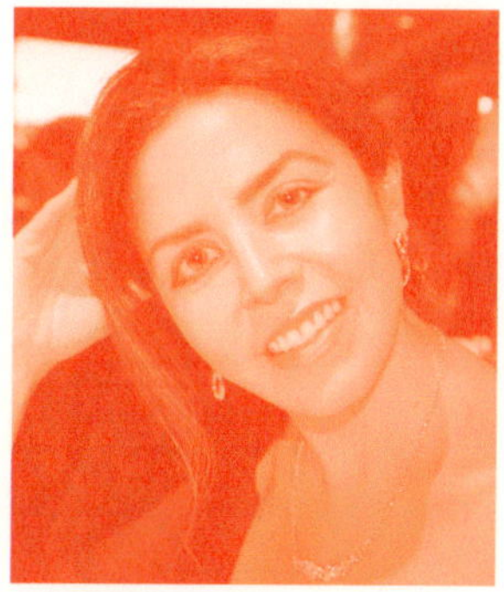

Supporting open minds since 2005

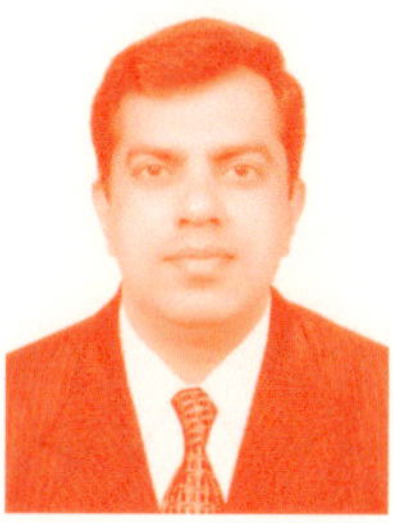
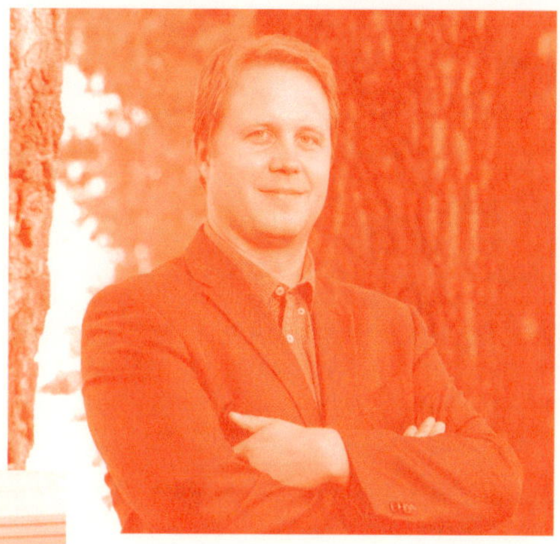
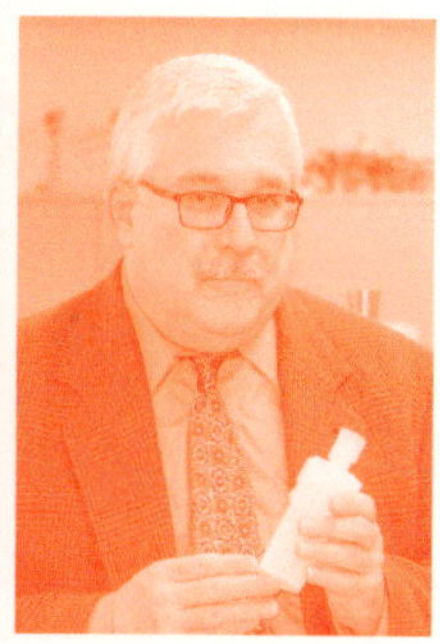
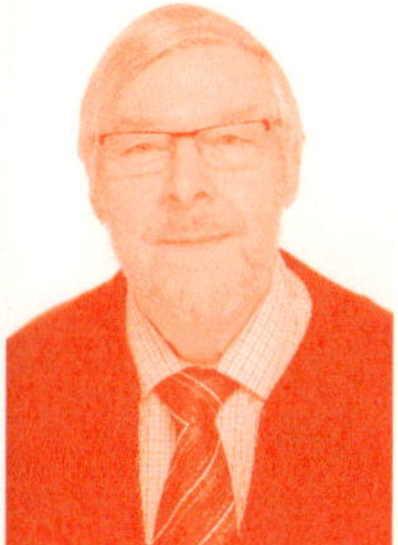
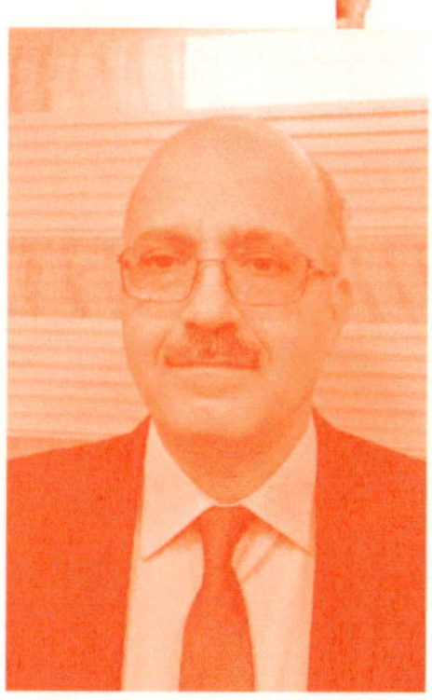
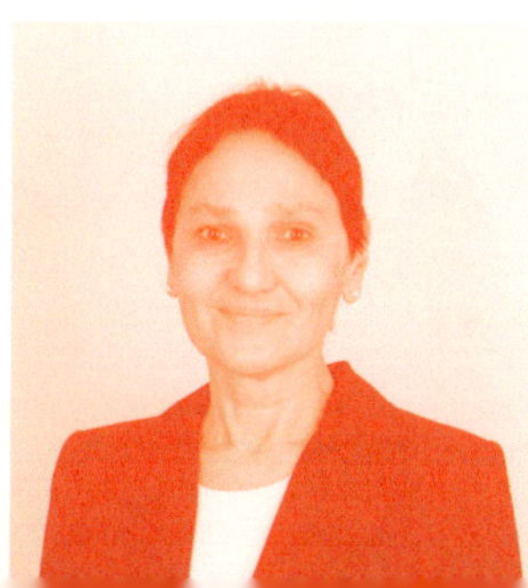
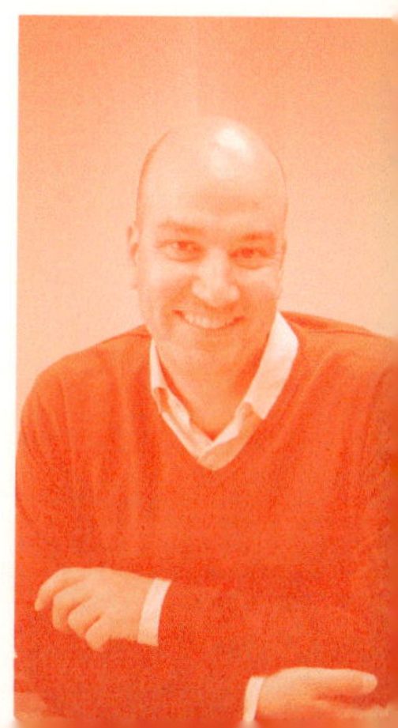

Vaccines - the History and Future
http://dx.doi.org/10.5772/intechopen.77910
Edited by Vijay Kumar

Contributors
Isaias Raw, Xiaoxia Dai, Yongmin Xiong, Na Li, Can Jian, Ericka N. Pompa-Mera, Mónica Salas-Rojas, Guillermo Galvez-Romero, Amaya Leunda, Katia Pauwels, Dulcilene Mayrink De Oliveira, Soraia De Oliveira Silva, Maria Norma Melo, Jonatan Marques Campos, Vijay Kumar

First published in London, United Kingdom, 2019 by IntechOpen
IntechOpen is the global imprint of INTECHOPEN LIMITED, registered in England and Wales, registration number: 11086078, The Shard, 25th floor, 32 London Bridge Street
London, SE19SG - United Kingdom
Printed in Croatia

British Library Cataloguing-in-Publication Data
A catalogue record for this book is available from the British Library

Additional hard and PDF copies can be obtained from orders@intechopen.com

Vaccines - the History and Future
Edited by Vijay Kumar
p. cm.
Print ISBN 978-1-78923-803-7
Online ISBN 978-1-78923-804-4
eBook (PDF) ISBN 978-1-83880-046-8

For EU product safety concerns:
IN TECH d.o.o., Prolaz Marije Krucifikse Kozulić 3, 51000 Rijeka, Croatia, info@intechopen.com or visit our website at intechopen.com.

Meet the editor

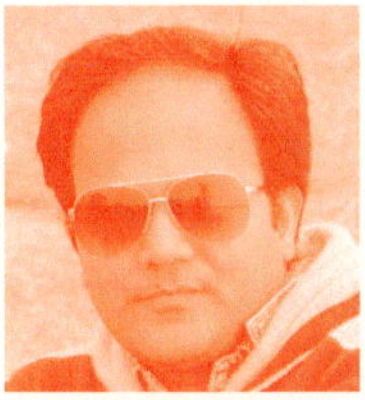

Dr. Vijay Kumar (PhD) has more than 15 years of research experience in the field of bacterial infections, including sepsis and pneumonia, innate immunity, immunopharmacology, immunomodulation, and inflammation. He completed his PhD in June 2009 from the Department of Microbiology, Panjab University, Chandigarh, India. Thereafter, he moved internationally and worked as a postdoctoral researcher at various hospitals and universities in Canada: Sainte-Justine Hospital, University de Montreal, Montreal, Quebec (2009–2010), Queen's University, Kingston, Ontario (2010–2012), and Sunnybrook Health Science Centre, University of Toronto, Toronto, Ontario (2012–2013). He also worked with the translational immunology group at Trinity College, Dublin, Ireland (2014–2015) before taking his current position working with the Children Health Clinical Unit, Faculty of Medicine, at the University of Queensland, Brisbane, Queensland, Australia. Dr. Kumar is the recipient of the prestigious "Piero Periti review article award" for 2008, awarded by the *Journal of Chemotherapy* in the field of immunomodulation and antimicrobials for the article entitled "Innate immunity in sepsis pathogenesis and its modulation: new immunomodulatory targets revealed." He was the recipient of a junior research and senior research fellowship (2004–2009) offered by the Indian Council for Medical Research, New Delhi, India. He has been awarded 17 travel awards to attend various international conferences in the field of infection and immunity. So far, he has published 50 publications in peer-reviewed international journals in this field. He also serves as an invited reviewer for journals like *Scientific Reports*, *British Journal of Pharmacology*, *Pharmacological Reports*, *Cellular and Molecular Immunology*, *Immunology*, *Innate Immunity*, etc.

Contents

Preface

Vaccines are quintessential for humankind as a preventive approach to eradicate the burden of infectious diseases. For example, certain sexually transmitted diseases (syphilis, gonorrhea, HIV-1 infection or acquired immunodeficiency syndrome, and trichomoniasis (a parasitic infection of the reproductive tract)), tuberculosis, acute respiratory infections, diarrheal diseases, certain parasitic infections (malaria, leishmaniasis, schistosomiasis, etc.), infections such as influenza, Ebola, Hanta, and Zika virus infections, and reemergence of certain infections, including measles, pertussis, or whooping cough, are possible global threats to humankind. The only possible preventive way to control these infections is through the development of effective vaccines. In addition to infectious diseases, these days development of vaccines as a tool to target cancer has also become an essential immunotherapeutic approach. Thus, vaccines are crucial tools to prevent these diseases all over the world. This book is an attempt to provide updated information required by researchers in the field of vaccinology. Following the Introduction section, the second chapter provides information regarding the scenario of innovation and development of new vaccines in developing countries. The third chapter is intended to provide updated information on types of vaccine and their development and role to target different infectious diseases. Furthermore, the fourth chapter is an informative chapter on regulatory aspects of genetically modified viral vectors and genetically modified organism-based vaccines. The fifth chapter gives emphasis to developing vaccination strategies against wildlife reservoirs for zoonotic viral infections (rabies, Hantavirus infection, and hepatitis E virus) in humans. The sixth and last chapter describes the development of vaccinia virus vectors to develop vaccines against leishmaniasis, a major health problem in developing countries. Thus, this book is a collection of well-written chapters by authors known in the field of vaccinology and immunology. However, the field of vaccinology and immunology is continuously changing and certain viewpoints expressed by the writers in this book may differ from other established scientists in the field. Therefore, I will ask readers to take this into consideration and follow developments and advancements in the field of vaccinology and immunology at both basic and clinical science levels.

Dr. Vijay Kumar, PhD
Research Fellow/Lecturer
Children Health Clinical Unit Queensland,
Faculty of Medicine,
The University of Queensland,
Brisbane, Australia

Section 1

History and Introduction of Vaccines

Chapter 1

Introductory Chapter: The Journey of Vaccines - The Past and the Present

Kumar Vijay

1. Introduction

The history of the process of vaccination and the concept to vaccinate is 1000 of year old (>3000 years) that originated in the ancient Indian peninsula (Northern and Eastern India) as a practice of variolation/inoculation (the immunization of individuals from the materials taken from the infected person) by "Woodiah" (Oriya) Brahmans since "time immemorial" due to its unidentifiable time of origin [1]. The evidence of protective measures of the process of variolation/inoculation is greatly described in the ancient Sanskrit text called Sacteya, mainly devoted to Dhanwantari, the physician [2]. Thereafter that technique may have spread to the China due to the transfer of education and knowledge as Chinese scholars were visiting the world's oldest Universities (Nalanda and Takshashila Vishwavidyalaya or University). Hence the technique of variolation moved from ancient India to the China around 1000 CE. Thereafter, the technique of variolation traveled to Africa and Turkey before its arrival to the European and American continents. Before the introduction of variolation there was no protective measure to counter the attack of smallpox and the observation was made by the Greek historian Thucydides (430 BC) that the attack of smallpox provides protection to the person surviving the attack of the smallpox. Evidence indicate the first existence of smallpox as a disease in ancient Egypt that reveled to ancient India through Egyptian traders visiting India during first millennia BC [3]. From India then it traveled to China in first century AD and reached in Japan in the sixth century AD [3]. It spread to Europe in the eleventh and twelfth centuries from there to North America (seventeenth century) and Australia (eighteenth century).

It is well established that smallpox is neither described in the Old and New Testaments nor in the classical Greek (including the Hippocratic and Galanus writings) and Roman literatures [2]. It was Abu Bakr Muhammad Ibn Zakariya al-Razi (864–930 CE), a Tehran (Iran) born Muslim physician who first differentiated between smallpox and the measles based on their symptoms and clinical examination of the patients [4]. However, the term smallpox is an English term for the disease, introduced first in India during the British rule and before it was known as the Masurika (For about 2000 years as mentioned in Charak and Sushruta Samhita before the Christian era) Basanta roga (*Paproga, Sitalika, Sitala, Gunri*, and *Guli*) or the spring disease in Eastern India. The concept of variolation or inoculation moved from India to the England in the early eighteenth century or 1721 by the British Lady Mary Wortley Montagu, who was living in Ottoman Empire (1716–1718) and communicated to her friend in Britain (Miss Sarah Chiswell, who died of smallpox 9 years later) about this technique by letters [2, 5]. Even in 1731 one British called Robert Coult in Bengal wrote a letter to Dr. Oliver Coult in England describing the procedure of variolation used in India to protect the local population from smallpox [6]. Dr. Edward Ives (1773), a British naval surgeon, also observed the procedure of variolation as described by the Robert Coult on his visit to India (Bengal) in 1755 [6]. Before the introduction of variolation/inoculation in England in the sixteenth century the burden of infectious diseases including smallpox, measles, whooping cough, dysentery, scarlet fever, influenza, and pneumonia accounted for the death of more than 30% children of age below 15 years as the record. The concept of variolation/inoculation was introduced in North America in 1721. By 1777, George Washington, ordered that all the soldiers and recruits of his army should be inoculated/variolated. Thus introduction of the concept of variolation was the first step towards the development of Edward Jenner's cowpox/smallpox vaccine, modern day vaccines, and the introduction of the concept of vaccination to fight against infectious diseases.

Almost all text books of immunology and microbiology mention Edward Jenner as a father of immunology or vaccination due to his invention of the technique called vaccination as he injected the cowpox immunogenic material (pus) isolated from the hand of Sarah Nelmes (a female milkmaid, who got the cowpox from the infected cow called Blossom) to the both arms of James Phipps (a young boy of 8 years) on May 14, 1796 [7]. However, the process of vaccination was developed almost 22 years before Edward Jenner by a farmer called Benjamin Jesty [7]. No one knows Benjamin Jesty. Even the reports are available to indicate the existence of the concept/Sanskrit literature of cowpox vaccine to induce the immunity against smallpox in ancient India. It may be an injustice to the real discoverer of the concept of cowpox vaccination but the journey of vaccines and vaccination had started that never looked back. However the technique of variolation banned or made illegal in Britain in 1840 and the Jenner's vaccination was promote and offered free of cost [3].

2. The development of vaccines from early nineteenth to twenty-first century

The early eighteenth century saw development of the vaccination procedure against small pox and its promotion in England by offering free vaccination there. Its spread all over the world revolutionized the field of vaccination against several other infectious diseases. However, the scientific origin of vaccines took at least a century following the discoveries made by Robert Koch and Louis Pasteur generating the concept there are pathogenic microbes/microorganisms causing infectious. Pasteur initiated attenuation of these pathogens in his laboratory by different methods including drying, heating, and exposing them to oxygen or passaging them in different animal hosts. The first live attenuated vaccine was developed for Rabies in 1885 and was used to immunize a boy named Josef Meister bitten by a rabid dog [8]. Thereafter killed whole organisms were used to develop vaccine against cholera (1896), typhoid (1896), and plague (1897) [9]. In second half of the twentieth century oral polio vaccine (OPV, 1963), measles (1963). Mumps (1967), and rubella (1969), all live attenuated vaccine came out along with several other vaccines (polio (injected, 1955), a killed whole organism vaccine, Anthrax vaccine (a protein-based vaccine, 1970), Hepatitis B surface antigen recombinant (a genetically engineered vaccine in 1986), and hepatitis A (a whole killed organism-based vaccine in 1996) were developed [9].

In twenty-first century, human papillomavirus (HPV) recombinant (quadrivalent in 2006), live attenuated vaccine Zoster in 2006, HPV recombinant (bivalent in 2009), pneumococcal conjugates (capsular polysaccharide conjugated with the career protein) (13-valent in 2010) are developed. Furthermore the live attenuated vaccine for the dengue virus infection is also developed by Sanofi Pasteur in 2016 and is called CYD-TDV that is sold under the brand name Dengvaxia [10, 11]. This live attenuated tetravalent chimeric vaccine is developed through the use of recombinant DNA technology by replacing the PrM (pre-membrane) and E (envelope) structural genes of the yellow fever attenuated 17D strain vaccine with those from four of the five dengue serotypes [11]. However this dengue vaccine is recommended to the patients previously infected with dengue virus infection otherwise it may exert adverse effects during subsequent infections as their manufacture, Sanofi Pasteur. The vaccine is approved to use 11 countries including Mexico, Philippines, Brazil, El Salvador, Costa Rica, Paraguay, Guatemala, Peru, Indonesia, Thailand and Singapore [12–15]. The dengue vaccine has shown consistence efficacy in healthy adults of Australia and ready to go in clinics [16]. The vaccine has shown immunogenicity and safety during a 5-year study [17] A most recent development in the field of vaccinology is the clinical trial for the live attenuated vaccine for Zika virus vaccine at the Johns Hopkins Bloomberg School of Public Health Centre for Immunization Research in Baltimore, Maryland, and at the Vaccine Testing Centre at the Larner College of Medicine at the University of Vermont in Burlington. The clinical trial for Zika virus is sponsored by National institute of allergy and infectious disease (NIAID), USA. In addition to the development of vaccines for infectious diseases these are also to develop against different cancers through targeting cancer-associated neoantigens.

The major aim of the book is to provide the readers an updated information on the field. For example, the first chapter of the book written by Dr. Raw Isaias has updated the progress of regarding the innovation and development of new vaccines and their candidates in developing countries like Brazil. In the second chapter, Dr. Dai has provided a great information regarding the different types of vaccines that will be informative for undergraduate and graduate students along with researchers. The third chapter of the book provides the regulatory journeys of applications with genetically modified viral vectors and novel vaccine candidates already reviewed by GMO (Genetically modified organisms) national competent authorities in Belgium and in Europe. This chapter will be crucial for the readers interested in regulatory affairs for the vaccines developed via GMOs. In fourth chapter, author (Leunda Amaya) has given an emphasis to target the vaccination strategies wildlife reservoirs including bats, boars, rodents, and other carnivorous animals serving as reservoirs for zoonotic viral infections (Rabies, Hanta virus infection, and Hepatitis E virus) in humans. The fifth and last chapter of the book written by Dr. Dulcilene describes the development of vaccinia virus vector to develop the vaccines against leishmaniasis that is major problem for developing countries of Asia, Africa and South America. Thus the book starts with the introductory chapter regarding the history and present status of the vaccines along with the other chapters contributed by the authors known in their field. Thus book is intended to provide the current and updated knowledge in the field of vaccinology.

Author details

Kumar Vijay

1 Children's Health Queensland Clinical Unit, School of Clinical Medicine, Faculty of Medicine, Mater Research, University of Queensland, St. Lucia, Brisbane, Queensland, Australia

2 School of Biomedical Sciences, Faculty of Medicine, University of Queensland, St. Lucia, Brisbane, Queensland, Australia

*Address all correspondence to: vij_tox@yahoo.com

References

[1] Brimnes N. Variolation, vaccination and popular resistance in early colonial South India. Medical History. 2004;**48**:199-228

[2] Behbehani AM. The smallpox story: Life and death of an old disease. Microbiological Reviews. 1983;**47**:455-509

[3] Thein MM, Goh LG, Phua KH. The smallpox story: From variolation to victory. Asia-Pacific Journal of Public Health. 1988;**2**:203-210

[4] Band IC, Reichel M. Al Rhazes and the beginning of the end of Smallpoxal rhazes and the beginning of the end of Smallpox notable notes. JAMA Dermatology. 2017;**153**:420-420

[5] Lahariya C. A brief history of vaccines & vaccination in India. The Indian Journal of Medical Research. 2014;**139**:491-511

[6] Nicholas RW. The goddess Śītalā and epidemic smallpox in Bengal. The Journal of Asian Studies. 1981;**41**:21-44

[7] Pead PJ. Benjamin Jesty: New light in the dawn of vaccination. Lancet (London, England). 2003;**362**:2104-2109

[8] Plotkin SA. Rabies vaccine prepared in human cell cultures: Progress and perspectives. Reviews of Infectious Diseases. 1980;**2**:433-448

[9] Plotkin S. History of vaccination. Proceedings of the National Academy of Sciences of the United States of America. 2014;**111**:12283-12287

[10] Capeding MR, Tran NH, Hadinegoro SRS, Ismail HIHJM, Chotpitayasunondh T, Chua MN, et al. Clinical efficacy and safety of a novel tetravalent dengue vaccine in healthy children in Asia: A phase 3, randomised, observer-masked, placebo-controlled trial. The Lancet. 2014;**384**:1358-1365

[11] Hadinegoro SR, Arredondo-García JL, Capeding MR, Deseda C, Chotpitayasunondh T, Dietze R, et al. Efficacy and long-term safety of a dengue vaccine in regions of endemic disease. New England Journal of Medicine. 2015;**373**:1195-1206

[12] Gessner BD, Halsey N. Dengue vaccine safety signal: Immune enhancement, waning immunity, or chance occurrence? Vaccine. 2017;**35**:3452-3456

[13] Hss A-S, Koh M-T, Tan KK, Chan LG, Zhou L, Bouckenooghe A, et al. Safety and immunogenicity of a tetravalent dengue vaccine in healthy children aged 2-11 years in Malaysia: A randomized, placebo-controlled, Phase III study. Vaccine. 2013;**31**:5814-5821

[14] Villar L, Dayan GH, Arredondo-García JL, Rivera DM, Cunha R, Deseda C, et al. Efficacy of a tetravalent dengue vaccine in children in Latin America. New England Journal of Medicine. 2015;**372**:113-123

[15] Yauch LE, Shresta S. Dengue virus vaccine development. Advances in Virus Research. 2014;**88**:315-372. DOI: 10.1016/B978-0-12-800098-4.00007-6

[16] Torresi J, Heron LG, Qiao M, Marjason J, Chambonneau L, Bouckenooghe A, et al. Lot-to-lot consistency of a tetravalent dengue vaccine in healthy adults in Australia: A randomised study. Vaccine. 2015;**33**:5127-5134

[17] Capeding MR, Laot TM, Boaz M, Wartel TA, Crevat D. Immunogenicity and safety of a tetravalent dengue vaccine during a five-year follow-up period. Trials in Vaccinology. 2015;**4**:19-23

Section 2

Vaccine Development and Developing Countries

Chapter 2

Developing Countries Can Innovate and Produce Vaccines: The Case of Butantan in Brazil

Isaias Raw

Abstract

Since the introduction of vaccines, governments learn that they are the most efficient and inexpensive tool to avoid the spreading of infectious diseases. It resulted in the creation of public research institutes to develop new vaccines, which gave birth to the vaccine industry, that is, growing in size by acquisition of competitors, which estimate that in 2019 they will sell $58 billion, where developing countries represent 80% of the world population, submitted to be dependent of production and prices from large producers. Incapable or not willing to assume the responsibility to produce, accept to purchase vaccines in bulk for filling and labeling as "producers." Butantan, a public not for profit institute became the first producer of specific anti-venoms and anti-rabies sera. In 1985, Butantan Center of Biotechnology attracted 25 young PhD, which accepted to carry on inovations and technical developments, setting dedicated plants to produce vaccines at affordable cost, aiming self-sufficiency to distribute free through the Ministry of Health. This chapter describes problems and solutions that must be faced to produce vaccine at a cost that developing countries can afford.

Keywords: vacines control epidemics, developing coutries 80% of world population, developing countries self-sufficiency, Butantan from innovation to production, anti-venonms and anti-toxinas, encloses production plants, pertussis reduction by DTP vaccine, whole pertussis low in LPS, MPLA from B pertusis as adjuvant, MPLA adjuvant reduce ¼ influenza doses an price of vaccine, vitamines A,D,E, riboflavin as adjuvants, pneumococcus-PSAP3 reduce cost of pneumo vaccine, plasma fractions not for sale, lung surfactant saves neonatals

1. Institute Butantan—research, process development, and production

1.1 Antivenoms and antitoxins

Antisnake venoms were the strength of Instituto Butantan and its priority [1–4]. At the New York World Fair, Vital Brazil saved the life of an employee of the Bronx Zoo bitten by a rattlesnake, which induced President Theodore Roosevelt pay a visit to Butantan in 1915. In 1983, Butantan sera production situation was scary: venoms were collected from snakes and administered to horses. The horses were bled and their blood collected in rusted milk drums, precipitated with ammonium sulfate, concentrated using a dirty towel, diluted and kept in large bottles until they "mature," and covered with mold! Probable other developing countries producers used the same ancient manufacturing process. Changing the production technology was the first goal of a recent Ph.D. group of researchers supported by the staff from the production laboratories under my supervision (**Figures 1–6**).

The first idea was to replicate the milk industry profile, creating a "hands-off" fully enclosed system using large stainless steel tanks and an industrial plate centrifuge. After snake venom inoculation, horse blood was collected in a 7-liter sterile bag with anticlotting solution, stirred, and kept in a cold room overnight. After plasma been removed, the settled cells were isotonic saline solution suspended and transferred to a connected-enclosed-4-liter bag to be returned to the same horse, characterizing plasmapheresis process and thus allowing repeated blood collection at short intervals.

The separated plasma was submitted to a complex process for immunoglobulin purification, began by precipitation by ammonium sulfate, followed by filtration, pepsin treatment (to remove the Fc portion of immunoglobulin to prevent complement activation), heath treatment, addition of caprylic acid to inactivate lipid-enveloped virus, finishing by an ion-exchange chromatography, which also removes viruses and other microorganisms. After sterile filtration, the final product was tested for neutralization potency and formulated to guarantee efficacy and safety.

Along 1985 to 2009, the production of antibothropic, anticrotalic, antielapidic, antilonomia, and combined antiarachnidic with other antivenomous insects sera reached about 700 million vials. The technology and the enclosed system were the model basis for the production of antitetanus, antidiphtheria, antibotulinic, and antirabic sera for human use. The antisera are usually presented in 40–100 ml vials diluted with isotonic sodium chloride solution, to be administered intravenously. Vials are kept refrigerated, and the freeze-drying process started to be introduced to avoid losses. Butantan supplies the demand of the Ministry of Health and began to export antisera to Latin America, some Africa countries, India, and even to attend the request of some countries in Europe and Australia. It was an unusual experience in learning by doing.

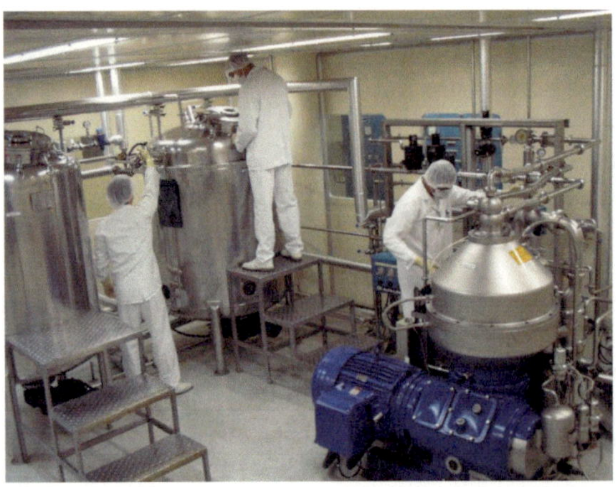

Figure 1.
Partial view of plasma fractionation production plant of antivenoms and antitoxins (Instituto Butantan Foundation).

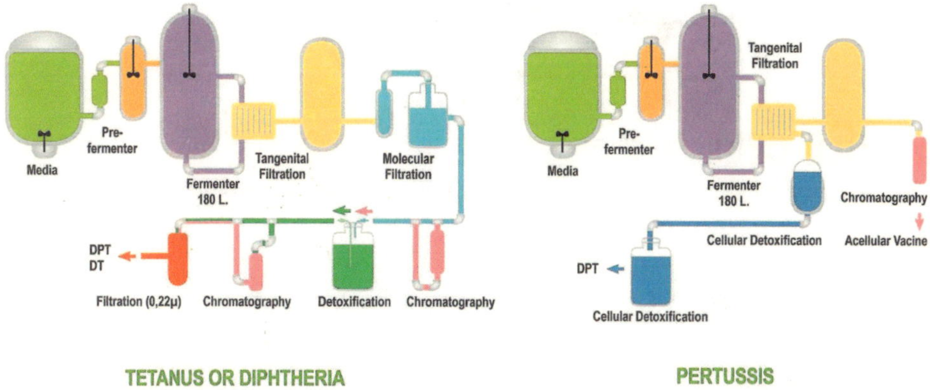

Figure 2.
Tetanus, diphtheria, and pertussis enclosed production systems.

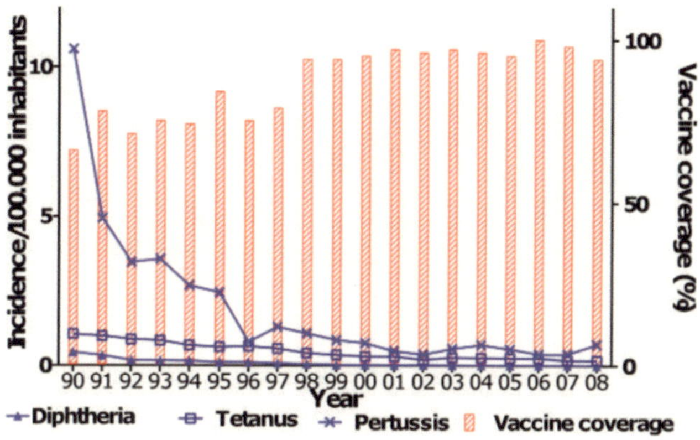

Figure 3.
Coverage of DTP vaccination and incidence per 100,000 inhabitants of pertussis, tetanus (except neonatal), and diphtheria in children below 1 year of age in Brazil from 1990 to 2008.

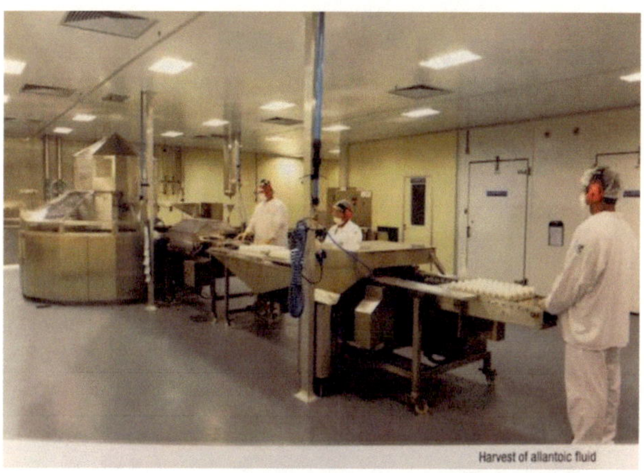

Figure 4.
Partial view of influenza production plant (Instituto Butantan Foundation).

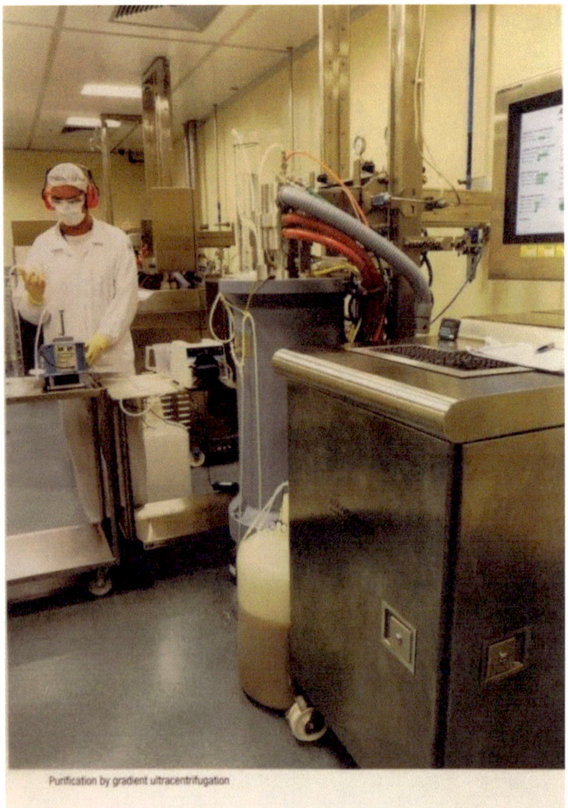

Figure 5.
Partial view of the hepatitis B production plant (Butantan institute foundation).

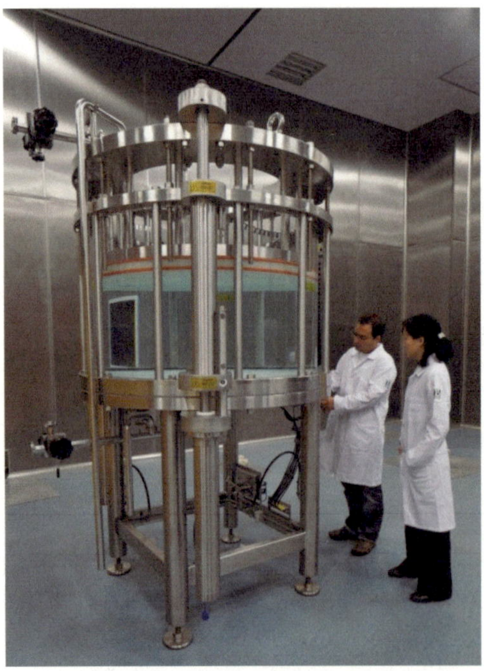

Figure 6.
One of the larger chromatography columns of plasma fractionation plant (Instituto Butantan Foundation).

2. Diphtheria tetanus and pertussis (DTP) vaccine

The gained experience in innovation, clinical testing, production development, and full production of antisera pushed our team to move next step into vaccine development, maintaining the dedicated enclosed plants, which guarantee hands off from the production staff [5–10].

The tetanus and diphtheria toxins production happened in enclosed large-scale cultivation systems as well as with the *Bordetella pertussis* strain (bioreactors 180–500 l). One observed particularity is that tetanus culture requires a vibromixer, a special device to promote the culture liquids shaking and not stirring. Bacteria were removed by tangential flow filtration, and toxins secreted in the media were purified by chromatography and finally detoxified basically following WHO recommendations.

A major concern was pertussis, a very common infant infection disease known as whooping cough. It can be fatal as a result of a variety of toxic substances from the classes of exotoxins and endotoxins. Among them, pertussis toxin, tracheal cytotoxin (that affect the respiratory epithelium), dermonecrotic toxin, and adenylyl cyclase (that inhibits phagocytosis) are the most studied and important.

We were able to select a strain of *B. pertussis* to produce an effective vaccine with mild reactogenicity and called it as whole cell pertussis (wP). After introduction of Butantan DTP vaccine (in between 1990 and 2009), the Ministry of Health reported that the incidence of pertussis infection had decreased from about 11/100.000 to 1/100.000, with practically no adverse reactions after vaccine administration. Around 70 million children were vaccinated.

The safety of Butantan's pertussis component of its DTP vaccine contrasted with the safety of DTP vaccine produced in Japan and in other countries. These vaccines are known as whole cell pertussis (wP). The development of an acellular pertussis (aP) vaccine based on purification of some virulence factors as pertussis toxin was a logical pathway. The acceptance of aP was achieved by most developed countries. These vaccines contained pertussis toxin, filamentous hemagglutinin (FHA), fimbria protein (FIM), and some pertactin. The aP vaccine required isolation and purification of all components, which raised its price from about US$ 0.16 to US$ 1.60, making it not accessible to the majority of the population from the developing countries. In 2013, CDC made a survey in the US and found that the aP confers a short protection, resulting in about 40.000 pertussis cases/year [11].

DTP vaccination scheme is usually carried out at 2, 4, 6, 18, and 48 months of age. One last booster occurred 10 years later. Thus, just for four DTP vaccine doses, replacing the DTwP by DTaP would represent an increase in cost of at least US$ 6.40 per capita, which is out of reach for poor countries. Even though a Brazilian publication [12] incited the use of aP for universal vaccination in Brazil at a "modest" cost of US$ 15,590 per life year saved, DTwP vaccination would cost 100x less.

There are other concerns for the use of aP [13]. Fetus and newborns may be exposed to pertussis infection before they are protected against it. Immunization occurs by three doses of DTP at 2–4–6 months of age. It is estimated that 45% of infant mortality occurs before they reach 5 years and is mainly concentrated before 6 months. This leads the idea to vaccinate pregnant women in the third trimester, generating maternal antibodies to be transferred to the babies by breast feeding. It is still necessary to fully investigate the safety of this type of vaccination to guarantee that there are no effects on the fetus [14–16].

Butantan has proposed an alternative for aP vaccine. It developed a process to remove the lipopolysaccharide (LPS), the most reactogenic component of the outer membrane of most gram-negative bacteria, without breaking the bacterial membrane, producing a whole cell pertussis vaccine low in LPS (wPlow). This vaccine was retested at Nederland Vaccine Institute [8] and currently is under additional clinical trials, as required by the Brazilian regulatory agency, to replace wP in our DTP, without increasing cost. Furthermore, the isolated LPS can be hydrolyzed to obtain monophosphoryl lipid A (MPLA), a power vaccine adjuvant.

Other alternative for the vaccination of the newborn is BPZE1, a live genetically attenuated pertussis, developed by Pasteur-Lilly by inactivating pertussis toxin, tracheal cytotoxin, and dermonecrotic toxin [17–18]. This vaccine will be administered in newborns as a single-dose nasal vaccine. Its clinical assay is being proposed.

3. Hepatitis B

Butantan developed a recombinant hepatitis B vaccine by genetic engineering, based on the hepatitis B surface antigen (HBs) and expressed in the yeast *Hansenula polymorpha* with a good yield [19–25]. The vaccine was tested in adults, adolescents, and newborns with the cooperation of the Institute of Tropical Medicine, the Medical School in Campinas and Oswaldo Cruz Institute [19–22]. It was the first recombinant vaccine developed in Brazil, approved and accepted for newborns by the regulatory authority in 1997. A total of 260 million doses were produced between 1997 and 2009, delivered to the Ministry of Health that distributed to all States for free administration to newborns, children, and adults. No significant adverse events were reported. The potential use of hepatitis B vaccine or antibody to treat chronic hepatitis B must be explored in the future [23].

Other new developments have been planned like the vaccine association with the adjuvant MPLA to reduce its concentration/dose (at least by fourfold as some assays have showed). These results consequently increase the vaccine's potential installed capacity without increasing the vaccine cost. A new genetic construction to express the preS antigen (the N-terminal polypeptide in the large (L) HBs antigen associated with virus attachment to the host cell receptor and membrane fusion during entry) was implemented considering the about 10% of nonresponsive adults. The use of the regular vaccine and the preS vaccine to treat chronic infection was also considered, but it was not yet tested. The success of the regular vaccine to protect newborns postponed the materialization of the last proposal.

Recently, a study was conducted in Brazil revealing that hepatitis B is not the prevalent strain causing hepatitis, with variation in different regions. Hepatitis A represents 58.7% followed by hepatitis D and F (23.4%), while B, C, and G are minor[23-24]. In a world overview, B/C relation represents 60% [24]. It is estimated that there are 5.000 cases of hepatitis C. The Ministry of Health is trying to cure with a patented drug that inhibits replication of the virus, sofosbuvir combined with daclatasvir, at a cost of about US$ 9000 per patient. The Instituto Oswaldo Cruz is trying to market a generic drug for four times less. The right of the Brazilian Ministry of Health to be able to supply the drug for all is being questioned by the patent holders, although it was accepted during the AIDS epidemics.

4. Butantan legacy, influenza, and adjuvants

Butantan assumed a national leadership in vaccine production in 2007, with dedicated plants for diphtheria, tetanus, pertussis, and hepatitis B [26–32]. Going from the innovation all the way to production, Butantan provided the

Society's demand to control wide spread infections, delivering vaccines free of charge to all population at risk, at acceptable cost to the resources of the Ministry of Health.

The public memoir goes back to 1918 when the "Spanish flue" reported 116.777 cases in city of São Paulo and killed 5.330 people. Those who could afford or have family elsewhere fled the country, leaving the streetcars to transport bodies to be buried in common graves. Government and Society respected the translation of "innovation" into vaccines and sera, safe, and efficient. Developing and manufacturing vaccines were different from buying bulks from large companies to formulate, fill, and label as made in the other countries. This situation was named at WHO meetings, the "coca-cola" model: buy bulk, dilute, and label made in the countries.

With the few vaccines and antisera mentioned, between 1985 to 2009, Butantan was able to produce about 720 million doses of effective and safe vaccines, representing 80% of the vaccines really made in Brazil, receiving for this about 40 honors, medals, and public grants. This was made possible by creating Butantan Foundation, a not-for-profit body that could operate as a private organism, by passing the Government rules, which would make impossible to buy reagents, supplies and equipment, maintain or built new labs and dedicated production plants, hire, and trend in service, the staff, to operate the plants, without the constrains of public rules, which were not adapted to solve public emergencies.

The next priority was flu epidemic risk. The "Spanish flu" reached Brazil in 1918 killing about 35,000 people. US-Barda realized, as pandemic spreads, that the total world production vaccine plants against flu could not supply the demand for vaccines, as the virus serotypes change each year and stocks could not survive and be used for the next epidemics.

Butantan seasonal or pandemic flu first action experience was to set a pilot laboratory to maintain and replicate influenza strains certified by WHO and CDC for production, and to train the staff for produce. A control lab to test and certify vaccines was installed. The State and Federal Government granted 10 million dollars to build the production lab, ordered when possible custom-made equipment (like the machine to destroy the infected shells that was built in Brazil). A central formulation plant was constructed and equipped with a modern automated filling line, to wash and sterilize vials, fill cap, and label vials, with filling capacity of 28,000 vials per hour, containing 10 doses each. A second automated filling system was added to cover for all the vaccines produced. Flu vaccine was cultivated in fertilized chicken eggs and, after extensive purification steps, was transferred for formulation and filling. C. Merrieux (latter Sanofi) extended its help to Butantan, following the plant construction and installation, and inspecting to be sure of our suppliers of chicken eggs comply the rules established by WHO.

The first formulated vaccines produced were taken to Merrieux's laboratory to be inspected and tested for the demanded requirements of the European Community. Butantan transported the vaccines using cold trucks to the central stock of the Ministry of Health in charge to vaccine distribution to all the state centers, which transfer them to municipal facilities during vaccination. To attend actual Brazilian yearly demand, about 100 million flu vaccine doses are necessary and it is not an easy task to achieve. It took a few years until the regulatory agency approved Butantan's vaccine, while Sanofi assumed an agreement to meantime supply the vaccine in bulk for formulation at Butantan. We reached, in 2017, the production of 60 million doses of flu vaccine given to children, young adults, pregnant women, and people above 60 years or with special health problems, doctors and nurses.

About 5 million Brazilians live above the equator line and, by mistake, they received the same Southern vaccine, in the same date. It was clear that they were vaccinated after the top of the flu season was over, and they were not protected [25]. The solution was to use part of the year to produce Northern flu vaccine to supply the population in the North. As the sole production plant in Latin America (other than a Sanofi plant that provides bulk to Birmex in Mexico), the excess vaccine production should be offered to PAHO rotating fund, solving the demand of vaccine influenza for Venezuela, Colombia, and Central America (some countries use North and other Southern vaccines).

Butantan became interested in using adjuvants for vaccine production, if they would guarantee more vaccines doses using the same facilities and thus reducing their costs. The first attempt, in 2002, was to use a formulated vitamin A in oil as a potential adjuvant to DTP [5]. The production of flu vaccine allowed Butantan to look into adding adjuvants to reduce antigen/dose, increasing the plant capacity and reducing the purchase of fertilized eggs. A ready formulated adjuvant was offered by one of the large producers of vaccines, but that would give to this company the control of the Brazilian market. We considered formulating our adjuvant using squalene as a component, but the supplier advertised that squalene was restricted to competitors. Squalene plus tocopherol (adjuvant system ASO3) resulted in some cases of narcolepsies in Scandinavia and China, attributed to a deficiency of hypocretin secretion by hypothalamic neurons [27–28]. ASO3 comes in two formulations, $ASO3_A$ with 11.86 mg/dose and $ASO3_B$ with 5.93 mg/dose [30]. In our assays, testing vitamins as adjuvants [29], we also included and studied tocopherol present in several multivitamins sold over the counter, and known to be toxic to monkeys. We developed the production of *Bordetella pertussis* monophosphoryl lipid A (MPLA), as a byproduct of the production of the low reactogenic pertussis vaccine (Plow). This MPLA has been shown to be a powerful adjuvant. We also tested vaccines with vitamins as adjuvants, which are produced in large volume as nutritional compounds. Testing 27 adjuvant combinations [5, 31–32], we concluded that the most promising was MPLA with the classical $Al(OH)_3$ [33]. Riboflavin and folic acid may act as a bridge to mucosal-associated invariant T cells (MAIT) and the major-histocompatibility-complex-related molecule MR1 [34]. We tested riboflavin combined with MPLA and a trivalent influenza vaccine, and we found a high increase in antibody titers [31].

We found that addition of adjuvants to influenza vaccine allowed a decrease in the usual dose of 15–3.75 μg. The adjuvant addition increased the vaccine production by 4-fold per egg, for the four split virus: A H1N1, H5N1, H3N2, and even H7N9, a new serotype spreading present in the vaccine. We also developed a whole virus vaccine technology in 2010 [35], recently being tested by several large-scale vaccine producers. Whole virus represents more than double production of vaccine/egg, as compared with split virus, and may decrease production cost by a factor of 2-to 5-fold, which would make preventive influenza vaccination affordable to developing and poor countries. In the whole virus, nucleoprotein is present, and they activate toll-3, toll-7, and toll-9 receptors of the host cell, explaining the higher immune response, but also produces antibodies that cross react with hypocretin receptor 2, which will require careful investigation before whole virus influenza vaccine is approved. There are results suggesting that the role of vaccine adjuvants like vitamin A and E increases the IgG1 response as high as squalene. Vitamin D was shown to modulate influenza immune response [35].

Vaccine	Age	Produced by
Hepatitis B	birth: 1, 6 months	Butantan
BCG intradermal [BCG-S1pertussis]	birth	Ataulfo Paiva Butantan
DTwP + HiB [DTwPlow + HiB]	2, 4, 6 months	Imported Butantan
Oral polio	2, 4, 6, 15 months	Biomanguinhos/GSK
[Rotavirus]	2, 4 months	Imported Butantan-NIH
Pneumococcal conj 10 valente	2, 4, 6, 10 months	Imported Butantan
Meningitis C conj	3, 6, 15 months	Imported
Yellow fever	9 months	Biomanguinhos

[vaccine]: under development.

Brazilian vaccination schedule.

5. New vaccines under development at Butantan

5.1 *Haemophilus influenza B*

Vaccines against *Haemophilus influenza B* are based on polysaccharides. The technologies for the production and the conjugation of the polysaccharides with the carrier protein were developed by Butantan, from 2007 to 2012. It is ready to move to full-scale production [36–38]. This product will allow to simplify vaccination of newborns, by combining in a single vial a pentavalent vaccine, DTwPlow, Hepatitis B and H. influenza B, all produced with our own technology, which depends on building a GMP-dedicated lab for *Haemophilus* production, evaluating trials and registration.

5.2 Rotavirus vaccine

An agreement NIH-Butantan authorized Butantan to produce the pentavalent rotavirus vaccine. Butantan was the first to produce experimental lots for a clinical trial phase I, which was conducted with good results [39]. The phases II and III trials were not yet authorized by Anvisa, but opened for the GSK tetravalent vaccine, using Biomanguinhos as an importer. This occupied the Brazilian public market for about six years. A new vaccine trial comparing with the GSK vaccine was planned with NHI, but the previous Butantan board of directors and management did not act.

5.3 Dengue vaccine

An agreement with NIH allowed Butantan to start a pilot production of dengue vaccine. Trials at School of Public Health of Pennsylvania were successful, but the clinical trial of Butantan vaccine was delayed 2 years by ANVISA, while allowed Sanofi to test their tetravalent vaccine in Brazil. After two years delay, Butantan is conducting the clinical tests in different regions of Brazil, using pilot-scale vaccines produced by Butantan. Clinical tests about to finish slowed down by an unusual decrease in the incidence due to unexpected weather changes. Production plant building is about to be completed by 2019. Meantime, Sanofi vaccine tested in Brazil will not be used and was not approved by any other countries due to serious adverse reactions. Even so, the Brazilian State of Paraná purchased the Sanofi dengue vaccine, while Philippines sued Sanofi for its adverse events.

5.4 DTwPlow and MPLA

The production plants developing antigens diphtheria and tetanus were supposed to be renovated to comply with WHO recommendations and requirements by ANVISA. Thus, at the moment, the production has been stopped. Meantime, we invested in the development of large-scale technology for MPLA from *B. pertussis*, expected to be used as an adjuvant for influenza and hepatitis B vaccines.

5.5 Pneumococcal vaccine

To replace a mix of 13 to 20 serotypes of pneumococcus, Butantan developed a vaccine based on recombinant pneumococcal surface protein A (PspA) from three different strains, making production easier and less expensive [40–42].

5.6 Modified BCG

By genetic engineering, a BCG expressing pertussis S1 protein was obtained. It was shown to be more immunogenic than the regular BCG and more effective in a mouse model of bladder papilloma. With this, new BCG Butantan intends to perform proper human trials and return to produce BCG to take place at Ataulfo Paiva Institute that is closing its operation [43–47].

5.7 Rabies vaccine for human use

Rabies vaccine was produced by Butantan for many years, using basic Pasteur process and using suckling mice to isolate brains [48–49]. The rabies virus inactivation used an ultraviolet lamp. This type of production was abandoned as the Ministry of Health requirement was to immunize each year about 42,000 domestic dogs. A new process was developed using Vero Cell in a serum-free media, followed by inactivation, to be used in human who had been bitten by suspected dogs [48–50]. The production and control of this vaccine limit the production to a few producers, being an expensive vaccine. Butantan invested in a large plant to where production is expected to be transferred in 2019.

6. Other process and products under development at Butantan

6.1 Plasma fractionation

According to the Brazilian Constitution, blood cannot be purchased from donor, nor its fractions sold; thus, plasma fractionation must be a public not-for-profit operation. Butantan did not have access to the plasma, but developed a process for hemoderivatives obtaining from human placenta extracts, establishing technologies to separate a series of proteins at high purity. The process allowed to isolate and purify albumin, immunoglobulin G, and some enzymes of potential interest for medical use [50–54]. When we got access to bags of human blood, we developed the purification process of factor VIII [55].

Butantan has worked in the development of a modern plant, replacing the Cohn method by sequential chromatographic steps, thus avoiding denaturation of fractions with potential clinical use caused by ethanol precipitation. The State of São Paulo with a few other states collected a large part of the human plasma collected in Brazil.

The Government of São Paulo provided funds to build a plant and purchase special equipment. The plant was built and part of the equipment acquired. It was planned to be an automatized facility, and a company with expertise was contracted to design a computerized central of control system that would direct the simultaneous steps of the process. This has already represented a partial investment of about US$ 200 million, while we maintained a small pilot plant to test every step of the complete process for purification of albumin, immunoglobulin, and coagulation factors. The scientific project started at Butantan in collaboration with Pharmacia, which was willing to participate in developing a plant to process about 150,000 l/year, purifying about ten different proteins.

Among other reasons, the project stopped after Pharmacia was sold to GE, which lack expertise and did not have the same interest in this project, which could be transferred to other countries, and Butantan would open its plant to train operators. A second impediment became the interest of a few large-scale plasma fractionation foreign companies, which would like to process Brazilian plasma in their existing plants, where Cohn method was utilized to supplement final purification by chromatography. There was an old precedent trying to establish a plasma fractionation plant in Brazil, expecting to produce albumin to rescue wound soldiers in the field, who were participating in the Second World War in Europe. This did not happen, but later opened the possibility for installation of a plant fractionation by a known company, which did not test the plasma to produce albumin, spreading hepatitis B in Brazil. Recently, there was a negotiation to open Butantan plant for a public private partnership, legally prohibited by the Constitution. Meantime, Butantan developed a chromatographic process to isolate as a first step the factor VIII, following with the isolation of IgG to be used to control infections, which are more specific for the country [53].

6.2 Lung surfactant

Each year, about 150,000 newborn dies by suffocation few minutes after the delivery. Most are premature, too small, do not cry after delivery, and do not open the alveoli. This can be corrected by administering to the newborn a lung surfactant. We assemble a team of investigators, including pediatricians from the Medical School of the University of São Paulo, which helped to develop a process for isolation of natural lung surfactant from pig lungs in an enclosed system and test in unborn piglets just after cesarean intervention [56–60]. The project was supported by grants of FAPESP and by a large meat producer, which supplied the pig lungs. A multistate clinical trial was carried out in public maternities with very good results, including cases of meconium aspiration. These good results supported the drug registration by the national regulatory agency.

The process initially developed extracted the crude lung surfactant with the solvent trichloroethylene, which was removed and recovered by evaporation under vacuum. The final surfactant is then lyophilized. As a byproduct of the surfactant production, we recover aprotinin, used in the surgery to replace stands. The process of isolation of the lung surfactant was redesigned to use less trichloroethylene and guarantee full removal during freeze-drying.

A large company on meat market in Brazil showed interest in funding the new plant in Butantan and expects to distribute lung surfactant for free to other countries like Congo where 100,000 newborns die each year. In contrast with Brazil where most deliveries occur in maternities, the introduction of surfactant in some countries with untrained mid-wife may only administer the surfactant as aerosols using a portable inhaler. The use of surfactant aerosol containing tobramycin is in our agenda, to treat cystic fibrosis and to speed up the recovery from postinfluenza among elder people.

Not all Butantan's projects were successful, even with the partnership of important laboratories in advanced countries. This has been the case of leishmaniosis, which affects Brazil and many countries in Africa and Asia. Visceral and cutaneous leishmaniosis infect dogs and are transmitted to man by mosquitos. It is increasing even in the developed state of São Paulo. New antigens are also been studied.

Difficulties are being faced also due to the reduction of funds to research institutes and even the closing of international research institutions where the developing world could find scientific support.

Butantan has proven the feasibility of public production of good quality biopharmaceuticals in developing countries, contributing to world science and innovation, translating the research into affordable vaccines for the population.

7. Conclusions

The Brazilian Constitution defines as role of the State to provide public health, specially controlling the infectious diseases where a few cases can spread the infection as epidemics to the whole population. The most effective program is to vaccinate, which should be affordable to the Government and then available for all.

In the early developments, advanced countries' governments invested in focused research, by creating public institutes and recruiting outstanding scientists to solve the needs for public health. They innovate and assay their developments for efficacy and safety, which requires an additional step going from the lab into developing production technology, which lead those scientists to create large-scale production facilities to make biopharmaceuticals available to the society. This was not the role of public institutes, and soon, large companies were created to supply, not just the national market, but developing countries, which represent 80% of the world population.

Soon, the public health motivated scientists were replaced by managers that measure their achievements not by saving lives but by volumes of sales, not responsible for public heath affordability. In recent time, producers of vaccines invested in innovation. Many public research institutes lost government support and some international health research institutes are closing. Developing countries lost support to receive technologies and to train scientists, so that they would be dependent forever and could not contribute to knowledge.

This brief description of scientific and industrial developments to answer to public health priorities represents the efforts of members of Butantan to convert innovation not only in publications, but also in vaccines and other biopharmaceuticals at costs that the national public health system can afford. This is easy to state, but in most countries difficult to achieve. As Butantan was able to provide to the society through the government some vaccines and other biologicals at affordable costs, we became recognized by our population, while considered by the large industries in developed countries as a bad example to other developing countries, becoming a target to be absorbed by the international large producers, not to produce to the government but to receive bulk, fill vials, and label as local production.

Also, some of the few local producers in developing countries were purchased to be closed. Offers for a public private partnership were not real, as both parts did not plan to implement, as large pharma had no intention to transfer recent technologies, while the local public producers, to avoid efforts and responsibilities, replace local production by buying bulks at costs dictated by the real for local filing. The large vaccine producer changed the goals, in part by transferring the leadership from scientists at service of the society to skilled managers, which measure success in terms of sales and profit, imposing their politics to developing countries market.

Buying smaller pharma in developing world, in most cases does not represent local production at affordable prices, but simply removal of competition.

There was an attempt to buy Butantan production units. In recent years, the institution has been suffering political and economic interferences that led to an undue stop of most of the production plants, pretending to be for major renovations. Instead, functional plants were destroyed, while purchasing the vaccines from large pharmas, without any concerns for our population or to provide affordable vaccines for the Ministry of Health.

Rebuilding Butantan and recover the expertise of the staff are not easy tasks and will require major investment. For other Latin America countries to begin without help is practically impossible. An interim plausible solution is to use a large unfinished Butantan's building to house a joint Latin American biotechnology center, while its plants are recovered to produce and train younger graduates participating in innovation international team, how to produce vaccines and they could take back with them the technologies developed at Butantan and maybe share with us clinical trials, avoiding the present prohibitive costs.

We think Butantan must go on with its public mission recovering good early Brazilian health public experiences and efforts. The case of AIDS pandemic was emblematic. It was partially controlled with new drugs, which were denied to poor countries, until Brazil challenged the patent. Same thing is in process to be repeated with the drug for treatment of hepatitis C, sold for $US 9000/person. And many other health public problems must be considered as neonatal syphilis is back to Brazil, even though it could be controlled with penicillin G, the first antibiotic discovered. The reason for the lack of penicillin is that its price became so low that private pharma lost interest in producing, illustrating the need of careful public health attention and decisions.

Author details

Isaias Raw
Instituto Butantan, São Paulo, Brazil

*Address all correspondence to: isaias.raw@butantan.gov.br

References

[1] Raw I. Antivenons and Antitoxins. Instituto-Fundação Butantan

[2] Dias WO et al. Chromatographic purification of anti-venoms and anti-toxins. Memórias do Instituto Butantan. 1989;**51**:195-203

[3] Leite LC, Furtado MF, Correa TC, Raw I. Characterization of the snake venoms from seven Brazilian species of Bothrops by FPLC anion-exchange chromatography. Comparative Biochemistry and Physiology. B. 1992;**102**:515-520

[4] Prieto da Silva AR, Yamagushi IK, Morais JF, Higashi HG, Raw I, Ho PL, et al. Cross reactivity of different specific Micrurus antivenom sera with homologous and heterologous snake venoms. Toxicon. 2001;**39**:949-953

[5] Dias WO, Horton DSPQ, Cainelli Gebara VCB, Furuyama N, Risoléo L, Ferreira VRF. Raw I: Vitamin A as adjuvant to the mouse immune response to pertussis, tetanus and diphtheria vaccines. Biotechnology Letters. 2002;**24**:1515-1518

[6] Dias WO, Horton DS, Takahashi CM. Raw I: A *Bordetella pertussis* acellular vaccine candidate: Antigenic characterization and antibody induction. Brazilian Journal of Medical and Biological Research. 1994;**27**:2607-2611

[7] Cainelli Gebara VC, Risoleo L, Lopes AP, Ferreira VR, Quintilio W, Lepine F, et al. Adjuvant and immunogenic activities of the 73kDa N-terminal alpha-domain of BrkA autotransporter and Cpn60/60kDa chaperonin of *Bordetella pertussis*. Vaccine. 2007;**25**:621-629

[8] Dias WO, van der Ark AA, Sakauchi MA, Kubrusly FS, Prestes AF, Borges MM, et al. An improved whole cell pertussis vaccine with reduced content of endotoxin. Human Vaccines & Immunotherapeutics. 2013;**9**:339-348

[9] Higashi HG, Luna E, Precioso AR, Vilela M, Kubrusly FS, Dias WO, et al. Acellular and "low" pertussis vaccines: Adverse events and the role of mutations. Revista do Instituto de Medicina Tropical de São Paulo. 2009;**51**:131-134

[10] Zorzeto TQ, Higashi HG, da Silva MT, Carniel EF, Dias WO, Ramalho VD, et al. Immunogenicity of a whole-cell pertussis vaccine with low lipopolysaccharide content in infants. Clinical and Vaccine Immunology. 2009;**16**:544-550

[11] Allen A. Public health. The pertussis paradox. Science. 2013;**341**:454-455

[12] Sartori AMC, de Soárez PC, Fernandes EG, Gryninger LCF, Viscondi JYK, Novaes HMD. Cost-effectiveness analysis of universal maternal immunization with tetanus-diphtheria-acellular pertussis (Tdap) vaccine in Brazil. Vaccine. 2016;**34**:1531-1539

[13] Siegrist CA. Neonatal and early life vaccinology. Vaccine. 2001;**19**:3331-3346

[14] Estes ML, McAllister AK. Immunology. Maternal TH17 cells take a toll on baby's brain. Science. 2016;**351**:919-920

[15] Kochhar S, Bauwens J, Bonhoeffer J. http://www.gaia-consortium.net/ GPPEa: Safety assessment of immunization in pregnancy. Vaccine. 2017;**35**:6469-6471

[16] Poland GA. Pertussis outbreaks and pertussis vaccines: New insights, new concerns, new recommendations? Vaccine. 2012;**30**:6957-6959

[17] Mielcarek N, Debrie AS, Raze D, Bertout J, Rouanet C, Younes AB, et al. Live attenuated *B. Pertussis* as a single-dose nasal vaccine against whooping cough. PLoS Pathogens. 2006;**2**:e65

[18] Feunou PF, Kammoun H, Debrie AS, Mielcarek N, Locht C. Long-term immunity against pertussis induced by a single nasal administration of live attenuated *B. Pertussis* BPZE1. Vaccine. 2010;**28**:7047-7053

[19] Ioshimoto LM, Rissato ML, Bonilha VS, Miyaki C, Raw I, Granovski N. Safety and immunogenicity of hepatitis B vaccine ButaNG in adults. Revista do Instituto de Medicina Tropical de São Paulo. 1999;**41**:191-193

[20] Turchi MD, Martelli CM, Ferraz ML, Silva AE, Cardoso D das D, Martelli P, et al. Immunogenicity of low-dose intramuscular and intradermal vaccination with recombinant hepatitis B vaccine. Revista do Instituto de Medicina Tropical de São Paulo. 1997;**39**:15-19

[21] Oliveira MD, Martins RM, Matos MA, Ferreira RC, Dias MA, Carneiro MA, et al. Seroepidemiology of hepatitis B virus infection and high rate of response to hepatitis B virus Butang vaccine in adolescents from low income families in Central Brazil. Memórias do Instituto Oswaldo Cruz. 2006;**101**:251-256

[22] Luma EJ et al. Efficacy and safety of Brazilian vaccine against hepatitis B in newborns. Rev Saúde Pública. 2009;**43**:1014-1020

[23] Pol S, Nalpas B, Driss F, Michel ML, Tiollais P, Denis J, et al. Efficacy and limitations of a specific immunotherapy in chronic hepatitis B. Journal of Hepatology. 2001;**34**:917-921

[24] Lampe E, Mello FCA, do Espírito-Santo MP, Oliveira CMC, Bertolini DA, Gonçales NSL, et al. Nationwide overview of the distribution of hepatitis B virus genotypes in Brazil: A 1000-sample multicentre study. The Journal of General Virology. 2017;**98**:1389-1398

[25] Araujo NM. Hepatitis B virus intergenotypic recombinants worldwide: An overview. Infection, Genetics and Evolution. 2015;**36**:500-510

[26] de Mello WA, de Paiva TM, Ishida MA, Benega MA, Dos Santos MC, Viboud C, et al. The dilemma of influenza vaccine recommendations when applied to the tropics: The Brazilian case examined under alternative scenarios. PLoS One. 2009;**4**:e5095

[27] Miller E, Andrews N, Stellitano L, Stowe J, Winstone AM, Shneerson J, et al. Risk of narcolepsy in children and young people receiving AS03 adjuvanted pandemic A/H1N1 2009 influenza vaccine: Retrospective analysis. BMJ. 2013;**346**:f794

[28] Han F, Lin L, Warby SC, Faraco J, Li J, Dong SX, et al. Narcolepsy onset is seasonal and increased following the 2009 H1N1 pandemic in China. Annals of Neurology. 2011;**70**:410-417

[29] Quintilio W, de Freitas FA, Rodriguez D, Kubrusly FS, Yourtov D, Miyaki C, et al. Vitamins as influenza vaccine adjuvant components. Archives of Virology. 2016;**161**:2787-2795

[30] Garcia-Sicilia J, Gillard P, Carmona A, Tejedor JC, Aristegui J, Merino JM, et al. Immunogenicity and safety of AS03-adjuvanted H1N1 pandemic vaccines in children and adolescents. Vaccine. 2011;**29**:4353-4361

[31] Quintilio W, Kubrusly FS, Iourtov D, Miyaki C, Sakauchi MA, Lúcio F, et al. *Bordetella pertussis* monophosphoryl lipid A as adjuvant for inactivated split virion influenza vaccine in mice. Vaccine. 2009;**27**:4219-4224

[32] Precioso AR, Miraglia JL, Campos LM, Goulart AC, Timenetsky MC, Cardoso MR, et al. A phase I randomized, double-blind, controlled trial of 2009 influenza A (H1N1) inactivated monovalent vaccines with different adjuvant systems. Vaccine. 2011;**29**:8974-8981

[33] Kjer-Nielsen L, Patel O, Corbett AJ, Le Nours J, Meehan B, Liu L, et al. MR1 presents microbial vitamin B metabolites to MAIT cells. Nature. 2012;**491**:717-723

[34] Miyaki C, Quintilio W, Miyaji EN, Botosso VF, Kubrusly FS, Santos FL, et al. Production of H5N1 (NIBRG-14) inactivated whole virus and split virion influenza vaccines and analysis of immunogenicity in mice using different adjuvant formulations. Vaccine. 2010;**28**:2505-2509

[35] Rezaei R, Aslani S, Marashi M, Rezaei F, Sharif-Paghaleh E. Immunomodulatory effects of vitamin D in influenza infection. Current Immunology Reviews. 2018;**14**(1):40-49

[36] Takagi M, Cabrera-Crespo J, Baruque-Ramos J, Zangirolami TC, Raw I, Tanizaki MM. Characterization of polysaccharide production of haemophilus influenzae type b and its relationship to bacterial cell growth. Applied Biochemistry and Biotechnology. 2003;**110**:91-100

[37] Albani SM, da Silva MR, Takagi M, Cabrera-Crespo J. Improvement in the purification process of the capsular polysaccharide from Haemophilus influenzae type b by using tangential ultrafiltration and diafiltration. Applied Biochemistry and Biotechnology. 2012;**167**:2068-2075

[38] Albani SM, da Silva MR, Fratelli F, Junior CP, Iourtov D, Cintra FO, et al. Polysaccharide purification from Haemophilus influenzae type b through tangential microfiltration. Carbohydrate Polymers. 2015;**116**:67-73

[39] Luna EJ, Frazatti-Gallina NM, Timenetsky MC, Cardoso MR, Veras MA, Miraglia JL, et al. A phase I clinical trial of a new 5-valent rotavirus vaccine. Vaccine. 2013;**31**:1100-1105

[40] Figueiredo DB, Carvalho E, Santos MP, Kraschowetz S, Zanardo RT, Campani G, et al. Production and purification of an untagged recombinant pneumococcal surface protein A (PspA4Pro) with high-purity and low endotoxin content. Applied Microbiology and Biotechnology. 2017;**101**:2305-2317

[41] Rodrigues TC, Oliveira MLS, Soares-Schanoski A, Chavez-Rico SL, Figueiredo DB, Gonçalves VM, et al. Mucosal immunization with PspA (Pneumococcal surface protein A)-adsorbed nanoparticles targeting the lungs for protection against pneumococcal infection. PLoS One. 2018;**13**:e0191692

[42] da Silva MA, Converso TR, Gonçalves VM, Leite LCC, Tanizaki MM, Barazzone GC. Conjugation of PspA4Pro with capsular Streptococcus pneumoniae polysaccharide serotype 14 does not reduce the induction of cross-reactive antibodies. Clinical and Vaccine Immunology. 2017;**24**(8):pli:e00228-17. DOI: 10.1128/CVI.00118-17. [According to Public Med]

[43] Nascimento IP, Dias WO, Quintilio W, Hsu T, Jacobs WR, Leite LC. Construction of an unmarked recombinant BCG expressing a pertussis antigen by auxotrophic complementation: Protection against *Bordetella pertussis* challenge in neonates. Vaccine. 2009;**27**:7346-7351

[44] Christ AP, Rodriguez D, Bortolatto J, Borducchi E, Keller A, Mucida D, et al. Enhancement of Th1 lung immunity induced by recombinant

Mycobacterium bovis Bacillus Calmette-Guerin attenuates airway allergic disease. American Journal of Respiratory Cell and Molecular Biology. 2010;**43**:243-252

[45] Carlétti D, Morais da Fonseca D, Gembre AF, Masson AP, Weijenborg Campos L, Leite LC, et al. A single dose of a DNA vaccine encoding apa coencapsulated with 6,6′-trehalose dimycolate in microspheres confers long-term protection against tuberculosis in Mycobacterium bovis BCG-primed mice. Clinical and Vaccine Immunology. 2013;**20**:1162-1169

[46] Goulart C, Rodriguez D, Kanno AI, Lu YJ, Malley R, Leite LC. Recombinant BCG expressing a PspA-PdT fusion protein protects mice against pneumococcal lethal challenge in a prime-boost strategy. Vaccine. 2017;**35**:1683-1691

[47] Nascimento IP, Dias WO, Mazzantini RP, Miyaji EN, Gamberini M, Quintilio W, et al. Recombinant Mycobacterium bovis BCG expressing pertussis toxin subunit S1 induces protection against an intracerebral challenge with live *Bordetella pertussis* in mice. Infection and Immunity. 2000;**68**:4877-4883

[48] Frazatti-Gallina NM, Mourão-Fuches RM, Paoli RL, Silva ML, Miyaki C, Valentini EJ, et al. Vero-cell rabies vaccine produced using serum-free medium. Vaccine. 2004;**23**:511-517

[49] Costa WA, Cunha RS, Bolzan VL, Silva AC, Caporale GM, Chaves LB, et al. Immunogenicity and safety of a new Vero cell rabies vaccine produced using serum-free medium. Vaccine. 2007;**25**:8140-8145

[50] Bettarello YM, Cabrera-Crespo J, Ho PL, Carvalho A, Raw I. Purification of superoxide dismutase from placental haemolisate blood: A simple and efficient method. Biochemistry and Molecular Biology International. 1993;**30**:45-51

[51] Wolff P, Tanaka AM, Chenker E, Cabrera-Crespo J, Raw I, Ho PL. Purification of fibroblast growth factor-2 from human placenta using tri(n-butyl)phosphate and sodium cholate. Biochimie. 1996;**78**:190-194

[52] Maimoni Gonçalves V, Cezar de Cerqueira Leite L, Raw I, Cabrera-Crespo J. Purification of catalase from human placenta. Biotechnology and Applied Biochemistry. 1999;**29** (Pt 1):73-77

[53] Cabrera-Crespo J, Goncalves VM, Martins EAL, Grellet S, Lopes APY, Raw I. Albumin purification from human placenta. Biotechnology and Applied Biochemistry. 2000;**31**:101-106

[54] Grellet S, Martins EAL, Goncalves VM, Lopes APY, Raw I, Cabrera-Crespo J. An associated process for the purification of immunoglobulin G, catalase, superoxide dismutase and albumin from haemolysed human placenta blood. Biotechnology and Applied Biochemistry. 2001;**34**:135-142

[55] Cheng E, Jinzenji D, Lorthiois AP, de Carvalho RR, Tanaka-Azevedo AM, Raw I, et al. Purification of coagulation factor VIII using chromatographic methods. Direct chromatography of plasma in anion exchange resins. Biotechnology Letters. 2010;**32**:1207-1214

[56] Kubrusly FS, de Lima Netto S, Iourtov D, Raw I, de Araujo PS. A natural surfactant from pig lungs. Biotechnology Letters. 2000;**22**:1251-1253

[57] Wu YZ, Medjane S, Chabot S, Kubrusly FS, Raw I, Chignard M, et al. Surfactant protein-A and phosphatidylglycerol suppress type IIA phospholipase A2 synthesis via nuclear

factor-kappaB. American Journal of Respiratory and Critical Care Medicine. 2003;**168**:692-699

[58] Kubrusly FS, Iourtov D, Leme E, Raw I. Pulmonary surfactant protein A isolation as a by-product of porcine pulmonary surfactant production. Biotechnology and Applied Biochemistry. 2004;**40**:173-179

[59] de Cássia Dias S, Sakauchi D, Abreu PA, de Lima Netto S, Iourtov D, Raw I, et al. Purification and characterization of aprotinin from porcine lungs. Biotechnology Letters. 2008;**30**:807-812

[60] de Cássia Dias S, dos Santos FL, Sakauchi D, Iourtov D, Raw I, Kubrusly FS. The porcine pulmonary surfactant protein A (pSP-A) immunogenicity evaluation in the murine model. Open Access. 2010

Section 3

Types of Vaccines

Chapter 3

Vaccine Types

Xiaoxia Dai, Yongmin Xiong, Na Li and Can Jian

Abstract

There are several different types of vaccines. Each type is designed to teach your immune system how to fight off certain kinds of germs and the serious diseases they cause. There are four main types of vaccines: live attenuated vaccines; inactivated vaccines; subunit, recombinant, polysaccharide, and conjugate vaccines; and toxoid vaccines.

Keywords: vaccine, type, attenuated, inactivated, recombinant

1. Introduction

Vaccines are biologics that provide active adaptive immunity against specific diseases. Vaccines usually contain drugs that resemble the microorganisms responsible for the disease and are often made from one of the killed or attenuated microorganisms, their toxins, or their surface proteins, introduced by mouth, by injection, or by nasal spray to stimulate the immune system in us and recognize the foreign agents and destroy them.

There are many success stories in vaccine. The first vaccine, against smallpox, a disease that had killed millions of people over the centuries by British physician Edward Jenner in 1796 [1], was derived from the benign cowpox virus, which provided immunity to small pox. In 1980, following an historic global campaign of surveillance and vaccination, the World Health Assembly declared smallpox eradicated. In the nineteenth and twentieth centuries, scientists following Jenner's model developed new vaccines to fight numerous deadly diseases, including polio, whooping cough, measles, tetanus, yellow fever, typhus, rubella mumps, varicella, and hepatitis B and many others [2]. Rabies was the first virus attenuated in a lab to create a vaccine for humans.

The vaccine exposes humans to very small and safe amounts of attenuated or killed viruses and bacteria. When you are exposed to it in later life, the immune system will learn to recognize and attack infections. So you will not get sick, or you may be infected lightly. During the process of immunity development, the body produces antibodies against specific microorganisms and creates defense. The next time the person encounters that microorganism, the antibody prevents him from causing disease or alleviates the severity of the disease, regardless of the way that a vaccine is made.

Vaccines are the most cost-effective healthcare interventions known to prevent death and disease. A dollar spent on a childhood vaccination not only helps save a life but greatly reduces spending on future healthcare. According to a new study from the University of North Carolina at Chapel Hill, vaccination efforts made in the world's poorest countries since 2001 will have prevented 20 million deaths and saved $350 billion in healthcare costs by 2020 [3]. There are still numerous diseases causing globally significant morbidity and mortality, for which no vaccines are available. Millions of people worldwide die of malaria, tuberculosis, and AIDS every year, diseases without effective vaccines. This chapter describes the vaccine types now in use and that may lead to the vaccines of the future.

2. Different types of vaccines

There are several different types of vaccines. Each type is designed to boost your immune system and prevent serious, life-threatening diseases. Four types of vaccines are currently available:

- live attenuated vaccines;
- inactivated vaccines;
- subunit, recombinant, polysaccharide, and conjugate vaccines; and
- toxoid vaccines.

2.1 Live attenuated vaccines

Live attenuated vaccines contain a version of the living virus that has been weakened so that it does not cause serious disease in people with healthy immune systems. Live attenuated vaccines can be made in several different ways. The most common methods involve passing the disease-causing virus through a series of cell cultures or animal embryos (typically chick embryos). Viruses are often attenuated by growing them in cells that they do not normally grow in for many generations. With each passage, the virus becomes better at replicating in new cells but loses its ability to replicate in human cells. Eventually, the attenuated virus will be less able to live in human cells and can be used in a vaccine. This method selects mutants that are more suitable for growth under abnormal culture conditions and is therefore less suitable for growth in natural hosts. Therefore, when attenuated viruses are given to a human, they are not able to replicate enough to cause illness like they would naturally but will still provoke an immune response that can protect against future infection. Albert Sabin's oral polio vaccine and measles, rubella, mumps, and varicella vaccines are all achieved by in vitro cell culture passage selection clones. The poliovirus used in the Sabin vaccine is attenuated by the growth of monkey kidney epithelial cells. The measles vaccine contains a strain of rubella virus that grows in duck embryo cells and later grows in human cell lines [4–8]. Another live vaccine that has so far only been used in the military to prevent epidemic pneumonia includes adenoviruses 4 and 7 grown in human diploid cell lines and orally administered for replication in the intestine [9]. Other live vaccines that are attenuated in cell culture passages are attenuated monovalent rotavirus vaccines in Vero cells [10] and Japanese encephalitis virus strain SA14-14-2 [11]. Some viral vaccines are grown in chicken eggs; live attenuated influenza vaccine and yellow fever vaccines are currently produced in embryonated hen's eggs, a method developed in the late 1930s [12, 13].

Live attenuated vaccines have advantages and disadvantages. Live attenuated vaccines are ideal for teaching the immune system against specific viruses because they are closest to natural infections. They often require only a single immunization, eliminating the need for repeated boosters. And these vaccines are relatively easy to create for certain viruses.

The Sabine polio vaccine consists of three attenuated poliovirus strains that are orally administered to children in sugar cube or sugar liquid. The attenuated virus colonizes the gut and produces protective immunity against all three virulent poliovirus strains. Unlike most other attenuated vaccines that require a single immunization dose, the Sabin polio vaccine requires a booster because the three attenuated polioviruses in the vaccine interfere with each other's replication in the gut.

The main disadvantage of attenuated vaccines is the possibility they will revert to a virulent form and cause disease. These vaccines cannot be administered to people with weakened immune systems due to cancer, HIV, or other immune system depressing diseases. Attenuated vaccines also may be associated with complications similar to those seen in the natural disease. Live attenuated vaccines usually have to be refrigerated and protected from light. It can be difficult to ship these vaccines overseas and use them in places where there is lack of refrigeration. This technique does not work well for bacteria; therefore there are few live bacterial vaccines. The virus is very simple, but for bacteria, which have thousands of gene, is at least a hundred times larger than a typical virus. This makes bacteria more difficult to control and manipulate than viruses. Currently, scientists are trying to remove key genes from certain bacteria in order to create a weakened version for vaccines.

Immunization using this strategy are [14]:

Viral:

- MMR vaccine;
- *Rotavirus* vaccine;
- oral polio vaccine (not used in the USA);
- influenza vaccine (nasal spray) FluMist;
- varicella (chickenpox) vaccine;
- shingles vaccine;
- yellow fever vaccine;
- adenovirus oral vaccine (military); and
- *Vaccinia* vaccine.

2.2 Inactivated vaccines

Another common method of vaccine production is inactivation of the pathogen by heat or by chemical treatment. This destroys the pathogen's ability to replicate but keeps it "intact" so that the immune system can still recognize it. Maintaining the epitope structure on the epitope antigen during inactivation is critical. Heat inactivation is generally unsatisfactory because it results in extensive denaturation of the protein; therefore, any epitope that is dependent on higher levels of protein structure may change significantly. Chemical inactivation with formaldehyde or formalin has been successful. The Salk polio vaccine is produced by formaldehyde inactivation.

Because killed or inactivated pathogens cannot replicate at all, they cannot revert to a more virulent form capable of causing disease (as discussed above with live attenuated vaccines). Attenuated vaccines generally require only one dose to induce long-lasting immunity. However, inactivated vaccine tends to provide a shorter length of protection than live vaccines and is more likely to require boosters to create long-term immunity.

A vaccine consisting of orally administered killed cholera bacteria with or without the B subunit of cholera toxin has been developed [15]. Formalin-inactivated whole-cell pertussis vaccine was tested by Madsen [16], and later it was shown to be relatively successful in controlling severe disease [17]. In 1923, Glenny and Hopkins reduced the toxicity of diphtheria toxin by formalin treatment [18]. Ramon has improved this finding and has shown that it is possible to inactivate the toxicity of these molecules while retaining their ability to induce toxin-neutralizing antibodies [19]. In the twentieth century, chemical inactivation was also applied to viruses. Influenza vaccine was the first successful inactivated virus vaccine [20].

Inactivated whole bio vaccines still present certain risks, even if they contain killed pathogens. When formaldehyde failed to kill all viruses in both vaccine batches, serious complications of the first Salk vaccines occurred, which led to a high proportion of polio (poliomyelitis).

Inactivated vaccines are used to protect against:

- hepatitis A;
- flu (shot only);
- polio (shot only); and
- rabies.

2.3 Subunit, recombinant, polysaccharide, and conjugate vaccines

The first vaccine, the smallpox vaccine, consists of live attenuated viruses, but it does not cause disease in human hosts. Many of the vaccines used today, including measles vaccines, yellow fever vaccine, and some influenza vaccines, use live attenuated viruses. Others use inactivated forms of toxins made from killed form of virus, debris of bacteria, or bacteria. The killed virus, bacterial debris, and inactivated toxins will not cause disease but will still cause immune reactions and prevent future infections. However, new techniques are also being developed to make different types of vaccines.

Subunit, recombinant, polysaccharide, and conjugate vaccines are biosynthetic vaccines. Biosynthetic vaccines contain man-made substances that are very similar to pieces of the virus or bacteria. The hepatitis B vaccine is an example.

Since these vaccines use only specific pieces of the germ, they show a very strong immune response, which targets the main part of the germ. It can also be used by almost everyone who needs them, including people with weakened immune system and long-term health problems. Vaccines consisting of specific purified molecules derived from pathogens can avoid some of the risks associated with attenuated or killed organism vaccines.

One limitation of these vaccines is that you may need booster shots to get ongoing protection against diseases.

Subunit vaccines use only a subset of target pathogens to stimulate the immune system's response. This can be done by isolating a specific protein from the pathogen and presenting it separately as an antigen. Acellular pertussis vaccines and influenza vaccines (injected forms) are examples of subunit vaccines.

Another subunit vaccine can be created by genetic engineering. The gene encoding the vaccine protein is inserted into another virus or inserted into a cultured production cell. Vaccine proteins are also produced when the vector virus is propagated. The result of this approach is a recombinant vaccine: the immune system will recognize the expressed protein and provide future protection against the target virus. Many genes encoding surface antigens from viral, bacterial, and protozoal pathogens have been successfully cloned into bacterial, yeast, insect, or mammalian expression systems, and the expressed antigens are used for vaccine development. A hepatitis B vaccine that is approved for use in humans is a recombinant vaccine. The vaccine was developed by cloning the hepatitis B virus surface antigen (HBsAg) gene and expressing it in yeast cells. Recombinant yeast cells proliferate in large fermenters, and HBsAg accumulates in cells. At the end of the fermentation, recombinant HBsAg are harvested by disrupting yeast cells, which is then purified by biochemical techniques. This recombinant hepatitis B vaccine has been shown to induce the production of protective antibodies [21, 22].

Human papillomavirus (HPV) vaccine is another vaccine made using genetic engineering. Two types of HPV vaccine are available, Gardasil (marketed by Merck and protecting against types 6, 11, 16, and 18 of the human papillomavirus) and Cervarix (marketed by GlaxoSmithKline and protecting against types 16 and 18 only). Both are made in the same way: for each strain, a single viral protein was isolated. When these proteins are expressed, viruslike particles (VLPs) are produced. These VLPs contain no genetic material that causes disease but promote immune responses and protect future HPV infection.

Recombinant vector vaccines use attenuated viruses (or bacterial strains) as vectors. A gene encoding a major antigen of a particularly virulent pathogen can be introduced into an attenuated virus or bacterium. The attenuated organism acts as a vector that replicates and expresses the gene product of the pathogen in the host.

Baculovirus which is a virus that infects only insects can be used as a vector, and genes for specific immunogenic surface proteins of influenza virus can be inserted. Once the modified virus is introduced into humans, the immunogen is expressed and displayed, producing an immune response against the immunogen and producing an immune response to the immunogen from which it is derived. In addition to insect viruses, human adenoviruses have been identified as potential carriers for recombinant vaccines, particularly against diseases such as AIDS. *Vaccinia virus*, the attenuated vaccine used to eradicate smallpox, was the first used in live recombinant vaccine approaches [23]. This large, complex virus, with a genome of about 200 genes, can be designed to carry dozens of foreign genes without compromising their ability to infect host cells and replicate. Experimental recombinant vaccinia strains have been designed to provide protection against influenza, rabies, and hepatitis B and other diseases.

DNA vaccines consist of plasmid DNA encoding antigenic proteins which are injected directly into the muscle of the recipient. The DNA itself inserts into the individual's cells, which then produce the antigen from the infectious agent. DNA vaccines have advantages over many existing vaccines. For example, the encoded protein is a native form of the host and has no denaturation or alteration. Therefore, the immune response is identical to the antigen expressed by the pathogen. The handling and storage of plasmid DNA do not require refrigeration, a feature that greatly reduces the cost and complexity of delivery. At present, there are human trials underway with several different DNA vaccines, including those for malaria, AIDS, influenza, and herpesvirus. Researchers hope that DNA vaccines can produce immunity against parasitic diseases such as malaria; however, there is currently no human vaccine in use for fighting parasites [24].

Conjugate vaccines are somewhat similar to recombinant vaccines: they are prepared using a combination of two different components. The conjugate vaccine was prepared using fragments from the coats of bacteria. These coatings are chemically linked to a carrier protein which is used as a vaccine. Conjugate vaccines are used to produce a more powerful co-immune response: in general, the presented "fragments" of the bacteria do not themselves produce a strong immune response, while the carrier protein produces a strong immune response. This fragment of bacterium does not cause disease, but when combined with carrier proteins, it can produce immunity against future infections. The vaccines currently in use for children against pneumococcal bacterial infections are made using this technique.

These vaccines are used to protect against:

- *Haemophilus influenzae* type b (Hib) disease;
- hepatitis B;
- human papillomavirus (HPV);
- whooping cough (part of the DTaP combined vaccine);
- pneumococcal disease;
- meningococcal disease; and
- shingles.

2.4 Toxoid vaccines

Toxoid vaccines are made from selected toxins that have been sufficiently attenuated and are able to induce a humoral immune response. These toxins produce many of the symptoms of the disease. For example, diphtheria and tetanus vaccines can be prepared by purifying bacterial toxins and then inactivating toxin with formaldehyde to form a toxoid. Inoculating with a toxoid induces an anti-toxoid antibody that is also capable of binding toxins and neutralizing their effects.

Toxoid vaccines tend not to have a duration of immunity comparable to attenuated viral vaccines; therefore, toxid vaccines, like some other types of vaccines, may need booster shots to get ongoing protection against diseases. Revaccination (booster) may be required multiple times in a single year depending on individual patient risk factors.

Toxoid vaccines are used to protect against:

- diphtheria; and
- tetanus.

3. Summary

There are still the needs for vaccines against other diseases. Millions of people worldwide die of malaria, tuberculosis, and AIDS every year, among which there are no effective disease vaccine. The road to successful development of vaccines that can be approved for human use, reasonably manufactured cost, and effective delivery to high-risk groups is expensive, long, and tedious.

Researchers continue to develop new vaccine types and improve current approaches.

Acknowledgements

This work was supported by the National Natural Scientific Foundation of China (Grant Nos. 81673117 and 81573140).

Conflict of interest

We have no conflict of interest.

Author details

Xiaoxia Dai*, Yongmin Xiong, Na Li and Can Jian
School of Public Health, Xi'an Jiaotong University Health Science Center, Xi'an, Shaanxi, People's Republic of China

*Address all correspondence to: xxiadai@mail.xjtu.edu.cn

References

[1] Behbehani AM. The smallpox story: Life and death of an old disease. Microbiological Reviews. 1983;**47**(4):455-509

[2] Plotkin S. History of vaccination. Proceedings of the National Academy of Sciences of the United States of America. 2014;**111**(34):12283-12287

[3] Ozawa S, Clark S, Portnoy A, Grewal S, Stack ML, Sinha A, et al. Estimated economic impact of vaccinations in 73 low- and middle-income countries, 2001-2020. Bulletin of the World Health Organization. 2017;**95**(9):629

[4] Sabin AB, Hennessen WA, Winsser J. Studies on variants of poliomyelitis virus—I: Experimental segregation and properties of avirulent variants of three immunologic types. The Journal of Experimental Medicine. 1954;**99**(6):551-576

[5] Katz SL et al. Studies on an attenuated measles-virus vaccine—VIII: General summary and evaluation of the results of vaccination. American Journal of Diseases of Children. 1960;**100**:942-946

[6] Hilleman MR, Buynak EB, Weibel RE, Stokes J Jr. Live, attenuated mumps-virus vaccine. The New England Journal of Medicine. 1968;**278**(5):227-232

[7] Plotkin SA, Farquhar JD, Katz M, Buser F. Attenuation of RA 27-3 rubella virus in WI-38 human diploid cells. American Journal of Diseases of Children. 1969;**118**(2):178-185

[8] Takahashi M, Okuno Y, Otsuka T, Osame J, Takamizawa A. Development of a live attenuated varicella vaccine. Biken Journal. 1975;**18**(1):25-33

[9] Top FH Jr, Buescher EL, Bancroft WH, Russell PK. Immunization with live types 7 and 4 adenovirus vaccines—II: Antibody response and protective effect against acute respiratory disease due to adenovirus type 7. The Journal of Infectious Diseases. 1971;**124**(2):155-160

[10] Bernstein DI et al. Safety and immunogenicity of live, attenuated human rotavirus vaccine 89-12. Vaccine. 1998;**16**(4):381-387

[11] Trent DW, Minor P, Jivapaisarnpong T, Shin J, WHO Working Group on the Quality, Safety and Efficacy of Japanese Encephalitis Vaccines Live Attenuated for Human Use. WHO working group on the quality, safety and efficacy of Japanese encephalitis vaccines (live attenuated) for human use, Bangkok, Thailand, 21-23 February, 2012. Biologicals. 2013;**41**(6):450-457

[12] Frierson JG. The yellow fever vaccine: A history. The Yale Journal of Biology and Medicine. 2010;**83**:77-85

[13] WHO. Recommendations to assure the quality, safety and efficacy of live attenuated yellow fever vaccines. Technical Report Series 978 Annex 5; 2010. pp. 241-314

[14] Minor PD. Live attenuated vaccines: Historical successes and current challenges. Virology. 2015;**479-480**:379-392

[15] Holmgren J et al. An oral B subunit-whole cell vaccine against cholera: From concept to successful field trial. Advances in Experimental Medicine and Biology. 1987;**216B**:1649-1660

[16] Madsen C. Vaccination against whooping cough. Journal of the American Medical Association. 1933;**101**:187-188

[17] Sauer LW. Whooping cough: Prevention and treatment. The Medical Clinics of North America. 1946;**30**:45-59

[18] Glenny AT, Hopkins BE. Diphtheria toxoid as an immunizing agent. British Journal of Experimental Pathology. 1923;**4**:283-288

[19] Ramon C. Sur le pouvoir floculant et sur les propriétés immunisantes d'une toxine diphthérique rendu anatoxique. Comptes Rendus de l'Académie des Sciences. 1923;**177**:1338-1340

[20] Francis T Jr, Magil TP. Vaccination of human subjects with virus of human influenza. Proceedings of the Society for Experimental Biology and Medicine. 1936;**33**:604-606

[21] World Health Organization. Hepatitis B vaccines: WHO position paper—recommendations. Vaccine. 2010;**28**:589-590

[22] World Health Organization. Global health sector strategy on Viral hepatitis 2016-2021. Towards ending viral hepatitis. WHO/HIV/2016.06

[23] Plotkin S, Mortimer E. Vaccines. New York: Harper Perennial; 1988

[24] Jaurigue JA, Seeberger PH. Parasite carbohydrate vaccines. Front Cell Infect Microbiology. 2017;7:248

Section 4

Targeting Zoonotic Diseases via Vaccination

Chapter 4

Vaccines Targeted to Zoonotic Viral Infections in the Wildlife: Potentials, Limitations, and Future Directions

Salas-Rojas Mónica, Gálvez-Romero Guillermo and Pompa-Mera Ericka Nelly

Abstract

Currently, emerging viruses such as arboviruses, flaviviruses, filovirus, and *orthohepeviruses* are important agents of emerging zoonoses in public health, because their cycles are maintained in the nature or wildlife, involving hematophagous arthropod vectors and a wide range of vertebrate hosts as the bats. Development of blocking-transmission vaccines against these emerging viruses in wildlife will allow disease control at the veterinary field, preventing emerging human viral infections.

Keywords: vaccines, HEV, hantavirus, RABV, wildlife

1. Introduction

Emerging and/or re-emerging zoonotic viral infections affect significantly the human health in many geographic areas of the world, highlighting their potential to spread from animal reservoirs and their ability to evolve their virulence properties. While the transmission of viruses from wild animal species to human is intermittent or rare, vaccines against zoonotic viral infections should be focused in wildlife reservoirs in order to prevent human disease.

In this chapter, we will focus on the vaccination in wildlife reservoirs, such as bats, rodents, boars, and carnivores, which play an important role in transmission of three emerging zoonotic viruses, rabies virus (RABV), hantavirus, and hepatitis E virus (HEV), to domestic species and humans.

We discuss the main challenges for efficacy improvement of vaccines, considering the diversity of viral *quasispecies* and antigenic and immunogenicity variations, as well as the biosafety and logistic problems associated to the delivery systems in the wildlife scenery. Finally, other emerging lethal viruses and the current approach to the development of vaccines will be discussed.

2. Hantavirus

Hantaviruses belong to family *Bunyaviridae*; they are enveloped viruses and have a negative-sense RNA organized in three segments denoted as small (S), medium (M), and large (L) [1, 2]. Unlike the other genera in the family, the hantaviruses are not transmitted by arthropods; their hosts are rodents and insectivores, and there is often an association of a type of virus with a host species [2]. In addition, new hantaviruses have been described in moles and shrews, as well as in bats, which increases the host range [3, 4]. Hantaviruses are maintained in rodent populations asymptomatic. Human infections are accidental (spillover), since for epidemiology and/or virus transmission cycle, the latter are a dead end (except for the case of Andes virus, where human-human transmission has been reported) [1, 5]. Transmissions among organisms occur by aerosol exposure, either by urine, feces, or saliva of infected animals, mainly [1].

In rodents, hantavirus infection has an acute phase (peak viremia) during first 2–3 weeks, with virus replication in target tissues and finally a persistent infection [1]. In humans, hantavirus infection can produce two presentations of the disease, depending on the type of virus with which it is infected: hemorrhagic fever with renal syndrome (HFRS) that occurs in Europe and Asia (Old World) mainly and the syndrome cardiopulmonary by hantavirus (HCPS) reported in the Americas (New World) [6]. It is important to note that HFRS can be caused by different viruses, the most common being Puumala and Dobrava in Europe and Hantaan and Seoul in Asia, while for the HCPS, the most common and lethal are *Sin Nombre* in North America and Andes in South America [7].

3. Vaccines against hantavirus

Currently, vaccine for humans approved by the FDA or any other institution for use in the USA or Europe is not available. An inactivated virus vaccine produced in mouse brain or in cell culture infected with Hantaan virus (HFRS vaccine) is applied in China and Korea. However, this vaccine may not be as effective against the other viruses that produce HFRS in Europe (Puumala and Dobrava) and not for those who produce HCPS (Sin Nombre and Andes) [7].

Considering the variety of hantaviruses and hosts, as well as the fact that there is no authorized or commercialized vaccine for human use that protects against all types of hantavirus, the development of a vaccine that can be applied to the natural reservoir (in this case rodents) is an option that should be considered.

When talking about vaccinating wildlife, the best option is the use of baits, which contain antigenic vaccine material, with stability under different environmental conditions. Since the capture and direct application of a vaccine would be unfeasible and the dispersion by a liquid or air (aerosol) constitutes a not selective administration, which might reach undesirable species and risk the risk of adverse effect, dispersion of the vaccine in species that had not been in contact naturally (in the case of attenuated vaccines) may not reach the desired species.

The viral target to which the vaccines are directed could be the Gn and Gc glycoproteins, which interact with the cellular receptor (integrins) for the entry of the virus into the cell [8]. We must consider the variability among the hantaviruses that can infect humans, since, as mentioned above, the vaccine applied in China and Korea runs the risk that, if it is not well designed, different vaccines against the hantavirus should be applied according to the region. Another point to consider in the design of this vaccine is the host variability that hantaviruses have as a group [6].

Mendoza et al. [9] described several characteristics desirable in the vaccine baits, such as having palatable baits for different species and stability of the vaccine in different environmental conditions among others. Development vaccine for animal use is faster in the process approval for commercial use. In this regard, the cost-benefit ratio is better, since the cost of production and distribution of a vaccine for veterinary use is lower, among other things [9].

The idea of One Health program, recently developed and adopted (due to the concern for all environmental changes that generate various human activities) [10], is the hypothesis that vaccination of natural reservoirs of host animals could stop the transmission of diseases to humans. Thus, vaccines targeted to wildlife reservoirs would affect the environment less and improve the health of the wild species in order to improve our health.

4. Rabies

Rabies is a zoonotic disease characterized by acute and lethal encephalitis, and it is caused by rabies virus (RABV), a *Lyssavirus* from *Rhabdoviridae* family. Rabies occurs after bites or scratches from rabid animal [11]. As a result of the increase in the human population (together with their companion animals) and the invasion of natural habitats and other anthropogenic activities, such as the traffic of wild species, there is also a high risk in the exposure to infectious pathogens coming from the wildlife. In the last decades, the knowledge of the diseases produced in wild animals that could produce spillover phenomena in the human population and zoonoses has been of special interest [12].

The majority of cases of rabies in humans are transmitted by dogs. It has been estimated that infection causes 60,000 cases per year, mainly in Asian, African, and American countries, [13].

There have been considerable efforts in vaccination campaigns in domestic fauna in the Americas, in order to control rabies virus transmission [13, 14]. However, wild mammals such as bats and carnivores play an important role in transmission to humans, particularly bats constitute the principal rabies reservoir in the Americas [15–17].

In Europe, during the 1960s, the only method used to contain wild rabies transmitted by red foxes was capturing and poisoning. However, it was an expensive and inefficient method in the long term [18]. One of the most cost-effective mechanisms to prevent the transmission of infection diseases is immunization. Since then, several approaches had been made for vaccination in the field with low effectiveness [18].

Nevertheless, the oral infection of mice coupled with the development of attenuated rabies strains gave the guideline for oral rabies vaccination (ORV) in wildlife [18–20].

Since the end of the 1970s, the ORV by means of baits was implemented in Europe using live attenuated rabies virus from 11 different strains, of which SAD Bern and SAD B19 were the most used [21]. This vaccination strategy resulted in the reduction of rabies by 80% and the eradication of the rabies disease in foxes in Western and Central Europe. In this regard, calendar of vaccination campaigns, the adequate distribution and density of baits, as well as the duration and follow-up of the ORV campaigns, were considered [21–23].

In the United States of America and Canada, the success story with ORV was replicated with the use of recombinant vaccines, employing the vaccinia virus (VRG) and a human adenovirus (ONRAB) that expresses the RABV glycoprotein [24]. In this case, the ORV programs were targeted at raccoons, gray foxes, and coyotes [25]. However, chiropters and carnivores are the main host of Lyssaviruses, and major spillover events have been detected from bats to carnivores [25].

As the European case, in Latin-American countries, the rabies control has been based in reservoir population reduction which means bat population reduction using anticoagulants [26]. Some approximations have been made for the development of ORV for bats taking advantage of the habit of constant grooming and close contact with other members of the population [27]; the recombinant vaccine is mixed with petrolatum paste or glycerin jelly and applied topically on the back of a bat vector [28–30]. These works are carried out in controlled environments with promising results, obtaining survival rates between 80 to 70% in *Eptesicus fuscus* bats and 70 to 100% in *Desmodus rotundus* [28–30].

5. Hepatitis E

Hepatitis E is a liver disease caused by infection with a virus known as hepatitis E virus (HEV), globally considered as an emerging public health problem [31]. While hepatitis E is considered as self-limited liver disease in humans, it can evolve as a chronic liver disease, whose complications are responsible for 44,000 deaths in 2015 [31, 32]. HEV infection can be acquired by fecal-oral route or contaminated water and other routes less frequent, such as zoonotic via ingestion of undercooked meat or meat products derived from infected animals, transfusion of infected blood products, and vertical transmission to fetus during pregnancy or occupational exposition [33, 34].

Since the first identification of HEV in 1983 [35], it was thought that the virus was only limited to animal species. However, in the recent years, an increasing number of HEV infections in humans have been reported [36–39]. Thus, and based on several anti-HEV antibody serosurveillance studies [37–46], it is important to highlight that the worldwide HEV prevalence seems to be higher than reported, as outbreaks or sporadic in pregnant women and immunocompromised patients [46–49].

This virus has a single, positive-stranded RNA genome of 7.2 kb in length. The genome contains three open reading frames (ORF1, ORF2, and ORF3). ORF2 encodes for viral capsid, which have immunogenic properties [50]. Hepatitis E virus is an RNA virus classified within the *Hepeviridae* family, belonging to the genus *Orthohepevirus* [51]. Four species are recognized. *Orthohepevirus A* viruses has been identified in several mammals, such as swine, wild boars, mongoose, camels, rabbits, and humans. In this regard, swine is considered the main reservoir, and the consumption of uncooked pork products has been associated with the disease [52]. *Orthohepevirus* A is divided into eight genotypes of HEV (HEV-1 to HEV-8). HEV-1 and HEV-2 genotypes can infect humans, while HEV-3 and HEV-4 have been isolated from humans, swine, and wild boars, being HEV-3 the genotype with the highest worldwide distribution [53].

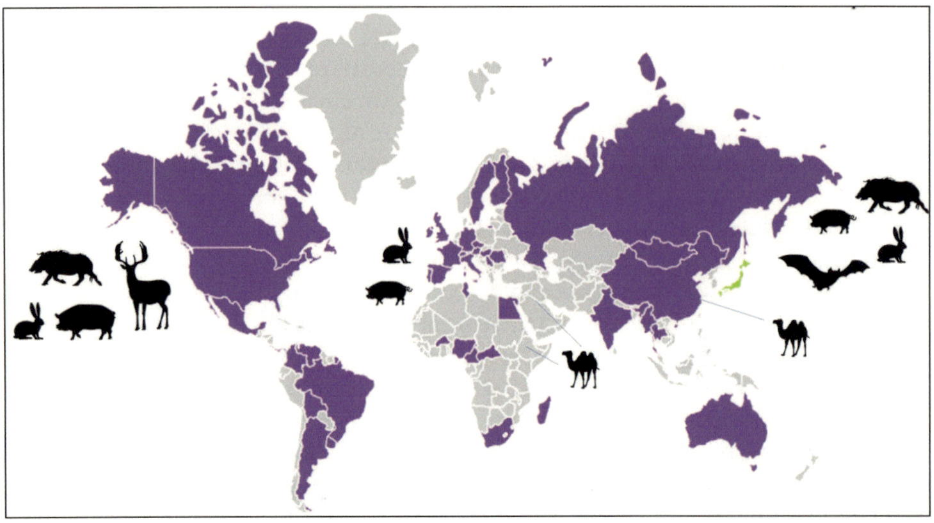

Figure 1.
Worldwide distribution of HEV and their reservoirs in the wildlife.

Genotypes HEV-5 and HEV-6 have been identified in wild boars, while HEV-7 and HEV-8 genotypes are isolated from camelids (**Figure 1**) [54]. *Orthohepevirus B* viruses infect mainly birds, *Orthohepevirus* C viruses infect rodents, and *Orthohepevirus* D virus has been restricted to bats [55]. Although a majority of species mentioned above are not in close contact with humans, some of them participate as intermediate hosts, thus causing infection in humans [56].

6. Vaccines anti-HEV

Vaccines represent the most effective prophylactic approach against several viral infections. Current WHO position considers vaccination against HEV [13], in order to prevent disease in high-risk groups such as pregnant women and immunocompromised individual. In this regard, anti-HEV recombinant vaccine, based on the capsid protein, was developed, showing efficacy of 88.5% [57]. In addition, a vaccine, anti-HEV 239 Hecolin (Xiamen Innovax Biotech), based in two epitopes from capsid (368–606 aa of ORF2), of genotype HEV-1, was only approved in China, with an efficacy of 86.8% [58, 59]. DNA anti-HEV vaccines have been developed (**Table 1**). In this regard, DNA vaccines have some advantages over use of attenuated viruses, besides to their stability at room temperature, making more affordable at veterinary field and the wildlife [60]. Thus, the delivery system for vaccination and genetic diversity of HEV must be considered in order to develop effective vaccines, especially in intermediate hosts such swine or wildlife reservoirs.

Finally, like the control strategies of wildlife rabies [65], the use of vaccine-laden bait delivery to intermediate hosts represents attractive alternatives useful to reduce the spread of HEV RABV circulation. While this approach is promising, it remains to be investigated.

Example	Immune response	Host	Reference
DNA vaccine ORF2 gene (1–660 amino acids, aa)	Anti-HEV IgG	Mouse	[61]
DNA vaccine based on HEV genes ORF2 (112–660) and ORF2(112–608), using papillomavirus pseudoviruses	IgG antibodies	Mouse	[62]
DNA vaccine based on complete ORF2 gene (1983 bp) in pVax plasmid	IgG-neutralizing antibodies	Rhesus monkey	[63]
Capsid protein/ORF2 HEV genotype 4	Anti-HEV IgG	Rhesus monkey	[64]

Table 1.
Experimental anti-HEV vaccines.

7. Zika vaccines

Zika virus (ZIKV) is an arthropod-borne virus (arbovirus), belonging to the family *Flaviviridae*, which was first isolated from a rhesus monkey in the Zika forest of Uganda in 1952 [66]. Since Brazil reported in 2015, the association ZIKV infection and microcephaly [67]; outbreaks and evidence of their transmission in many areas of Americas Africa and other regions have been reported [68]. Although ZIKV infection is considered as self-limited illness and minimally symptomatic for most individuals, it can be threatening for human health worldwide, in particular to unborn fetus [69].

Because arboviruses are often maintained in complex cycles involving vertebrates and blood-feeding vectors, not only humans are at high risk of ZIKV infection but also another species such as monkeys, domestic sheep, goats, horses, cows, ducks, rodents, bats, orangutans, and carabaos [69]. ZIKV infection has likely been present in bats since time. In this regard, anti-ZIKV antibodies with cross-reactivity to flaviviruses (yellow fever virus, West Nile virus, among others) were detected in bats from Uganda and Angola [70, 71]. Although it is unclear how ZIKV could circulate in bat populations, it is noteworthy that bats represent a competent reservoirs in wildlife, with potential for amplifying flaviviruses and, contributing thus in the sylvatic transmission of ZIKV [72]. In contrast, Bittar et al. [73] did not find serological and molecular evidence of past or latent arbovirus infections in captured bats from many areas of Brazil. Nevertheless, future studies are required to evaluate the role of bats as arbovirus reservoirs and to determine if these animal species are an important part of enzootic cycle of arboviruses [72].

Currently, there are no approved vaccines available to protect against infection. Unlikely to other antiviral vaccines, Zika vaccination must be approached mainly for the prevention of vertical transmission of the virus to the unborn fetus [74].

Finally, as long as a prophylactic vaccine is developed, it is important to consider that ZIKV is spreading rapidly into regions around the world where other flaviviruses, such as dengue virus (DENV) and West Nile virus (WNV), are endemic. In this regard, Zika virus is closely related to other flaviviruses, and cross-reactive antibody has the potential to exacerbate secondary flavivirus infections through antibody-dependent enhancement (ADE), leading to more severe forms of flavivirus disease [75].

8. Ebola and SARS-CoV vaccines

Ebola is a viral illness caused by *Ebola virus*. Five species of the genus *Ebolavirus* from Africa have been recognized, *Zaire ebolavirus* (ZEBOV), *Sudan ebolavirus* (SEBOV), *Cote d'Ivoire ebolavirus* (CEBOV), *Bundibugyo ebolavirus* (BEBOV), and *Reston ebolavirus* (REBOV), all belonging to *Filoviridae* family. Viral replication have a lethal nature, which involve necrosis of several lymph organs, kidneys, liver, testes, and ovaries; changes in vascular permeability; activation of the clotting cascade; and damage in platelets, among others [76]. Although the natural reservoir of the virus is unknown, it is assumed that bats represent a natural reservoir in the wildlife species, without causing disease [77], highlighting extensive coevolution of Ebola virus and bats, over time [76]. Therefore, feasibility of Ebola vaccine must focus on the prevention of Ebola in endemic areas as well as usage during sporadic outbreaks in humans [78]. Ideally, candidate vaccine must be able to confer interspecies cross-protection against SEBOV, BEBOV, and ZEBOV [76].

With respect to SARS-CoV, the development of a vaccine that is applied to wild vectors is a little more complex. Bats have been proposed as potential reservoirs, and there may be an intermediate host, such as civets [79]. However, there are still epidemiological studies that help us understand the dynamics of animals, *coronavirus*, and humans, in order to establish the best vaccination strategy, since not all zoonotic disease vector vaccination can be the solution.

9. Conclusions

Hantavirus, RABV, HEV, ZIKV, Ebola virus, and SARS-CoV are currently considered as emerging infectious pathogens to humans, whose reservoirs are in wildlife animals. While the transmission of these viruses from wildlife reservoirs to human is rare, it is important to develop control strategies in order to reduce the substantial impacts on human health and agricultural production. In several cases, such as rabies disease the vaccines targeted to wildlife reservoirs, represent a control measure friendly with the environment, in virtue of they help to the conservation of healthy habitats with available niches and wild prey for bats, avoiding the migration of these species to another areas.

Author details

Salas-Rojas Mónica[1], Gálvez-Romero Guillermo[1] and Pompa-Mera Ericka Nelly[2*]

1 Unidad de Investigación en Inmunología, Hospital de Pediatría, Centro Médico Nacional Siglo XXI, Instituto Mexicano del Seguro Social, Mexico City, México

2 Unidad de Investigación en Enfermedades Infecciosas y Parasitarias, Hospital de Pediatría, Centro Médico Nacional Siglo XXI, Instituto Mexicano del Seguro Social, Mexico City, México

*Address all correspondence to: erickanelly@yahoo.com.mx

References

[1] Easterbrook JD, Klein SL. Immunological mechanisms mediating hantavirus persistence in rodent reservoirs. PLoS Pathogens. 2008;**4**(11):e1000172. DOI: 10.1371/journal.ppat.1000172

[2] International Committee on Taxonomy of Viruses (ICTV). Available in: https://talk.ictvonline.org/ [Accessed: December 10, 2018]

[3] Guo WP, Lin XD, Wang W, Tian JH, Cong ML, Zhang HL, et al. Phylogeny and origins of hantaviruses harbored by bats, insectivores, and rodents. PLoS Pathogens. 2013;**9**(2):e1003159. DOI: 10.1371/journal.ppat.1003159

[4] Sabino-Santos G Jr, Maia FG, Vieira TM, de Lara Muylaert R, Lima SM, Gonçalves CB, et al. Evidence of hantavirus infection among bats in Brazil. The American Journal of Tropical Medicine and Hygiene. 2015;**93**(2):404-406. DOI: 10.4269/ajtmh.15-0032

[5] Martinez VP, Bellomo C, San Juan J, Pinna D, Forlenza R, Elder M, et al. Person-to-person transmission of Andes virus. Emerging Infectious Diseases. 2005;**11**(12):1848-1853

[6] Ermonval M, Baychelier F, Tordo N. What do we know about how hantaviruses interact with their different hosts? Viruses. 2016;**11**(8):8, E223. DOI: 10.3390/v8080223

[7] Schmaljohn CS. Vaccines for hantaviruses: Progress and issues. Expert Review of Vaccines. 2012;**11**(5):511-513. DOI: 10.1586/erv.12.15

[8] Cifuentes-Muñoz N, Salazar-Quiroz N, Tischler ND. Hantavirus Gn and Gc envelope glycoproteins: Key structural units for virus cell entry and virus assembly. Viruses. 2014;**6**(4):1801-1822. DOI: 10.3390/v6041801

[9] Mendoza EJ, Warner B, Kobinger G, Ogden NH, Safronetz D. Baited vaccines: A strategy to mitigate rodent-borne viral zoonoses in humans. Zoonoses and Public Health. 2018. In press. DOI: 10.1111/zph.12487

[10] Gebreyes WA, Dupouy-Camet J, Newport MJ, Oliveira CJ, Schlesinger LS, Saif YM, et al. The global one health paradigm: Challenges and opportunities for tackling infectious diseases at the human, animal, and environment interface in low-resource settings. PLoS Neglected Tropical Diseases. 2014;**8**(11):e3257. DOI: 10.1371/journal.pntd.0003257

[11] Lafon M. Rabies. In: Reiss CS, editor. Neurotropic Viral Infections. Vol. 85. Switzerland: Springer International Publishing; 2016, 2016. pp. 85-113. DOI: 10.1007/978-3-319-33133-1_4

[12] Gebreyes WA, Dupouy-Camet J, Newport MJ, Oliveira CJ, Schlesinger LS, Saif YM, et al. The global one health paradigm: Challenges and opportunities for tackling infectious diseases at the human, animal, and environment interface in low-resource settings. PLoS Neglected Tropical Diseases. 2014;**8**(11):e3257. DOI: 10.1371/journal.pntd.0003257

[13] WHO. 2017. http://www.who.int/rabies/epidemiology/en/ Available in: https://www.who.int/news-room/fact-sheets/detail/rabies

[14] de Thoisy B, Bourhy H, Delaval M, Pontier D, Dacheux L, Darcissac E, et al. Bioecological drivers of rabies virus circulation in a neotropical bat community. PLoS Neglected Tropical Diseases. 2016;**10**(1):e0004378. DOI: 10.1371/journal.pntd.0004378

[15] Rupprecht CE, Hanlon CA, Hemachudha T. Rabies re-examined. The Lancet Infectious Diseases. 2002;**2**(6):327-343

[16] Oliveira RN, de Souza SP, Lobo RS, Castilho JG, Macedo CI, Carnieli P Jr, et al. Rabies virus in insectivorous bats: Implications of the diversity of the nucleoprotein and glycoprotein genes for molecular epidemiology. Virology. 2010;**405**(2):352-360. DOI: 10.1016/j.virol.2010.05.030

[17] Allendorf SD, Cortez A, Heinemann MB, Harary CM, Antunes JM, Peres MG, et al. Rabies virus distribution in tissues and molecular characterization of strains from naturally infected non-hematophagous bats. Virus Research. 2012;**165**(2):119-125. DOI: 10.1016/j.virusres.2012.01.011

[18] Baer GM. In: Baer GM, editor. The Natural History of Rabies. Vol. 2. New York: Academic; 1975. pp. 261-266

[19] Hudson DA, Winkler WG, Sikes RK. A field study with an automatic inoculating device for wildlife. EIS Conf., Center for Disease Control, Atlanta, Georgia; 1968

[20] Baer GM, Abelseth MK, Debbie JG. Oral vaccination of foxes against rabies. American Journal of Epidemiology. 1971;**93**(6):487-490

[21] Müller TF, Schröder R, Wysocki P, Mettenleiter TC, Freuling CM. Spatio-temporal use of oral rabies vaccines in fox rabies elimination programmes in Europe. PLoS Neglected Tropical Diseases. 2015;**9**(8):e0003953. DOI: 10.1371/journal.pntd.0003953

[22] Pastoret PP, Kappeler A, Aubert M. European rabies control and its history. In: King AA, Fooks AR, Aubert M, Wandeler AI, editors. Historical Perspective of Rabies in Europe and the Mediterranean Basin. Paris: OIE; 2004. pp. 337-350

[23] Freuling C, Hampson K, Selhorst T, Schröder R, Meslin FX, Mettenleiter TC, et al. The elimination of fox rabies from Europe: Determinants of success and lessons for the future. Philosophical Transactions of the Royal Society B. 2013;**368**(1623):1-13. DOI: 10.1098/rstb.2012.0142

[24] Mendoza EJ, Warner B, Kobinger G, Ogden NH, Safronetz D. Baited vaccines: A strategy to mitigate rodent-borne viral zoonoses in humans. Zoonoses and Public Health. 2018. DOI: 10.1111/zph.12487. In press

[25] Rupprecht CE, Hanlon CA, Slate D. Oral vaccination of wildlife against rabies: Opportunities and challenges in prevention and control. Developmental Biology (Basel). 2004;**119**:173-184

[26] Linhart SB, Flores Crespo R, Mitchell GC. Controle de murciélagos vampiros por medio de un anticoagulante. Boletín de la Oficina Sanitaria Panamericana. 1972;**73**:100-109

[27] Greenhall AM. Notes on behavior of captive bats. Mammalia. 1965;**29**(4):441-451

[28] Almeida MF, Martorelli LF, Aires CC, Barros RF, Massad E. Vaccinating the vampire bat Desmodus rotundus against rabies. Virus Research. 2008;**137**(2):275-277. DOI: 10.1016/j.virusres.2008.07.024

[29] Stading B, Ellison JA, Carson WC, Satheshkumar PS, Rocke TE, Osorio JE. Protection of bats (*Eptesicus fuscus*) against rabies following topical or oronasal exposure to a recombinant raccoon poxvirus vaccine. PLoS Neglected Tropical Diseases. 2017;**11**(10):e0005958. DOI: 10.1371/journal.pntd.0005958

[30] Escobar LE, Peterson AT, Favi M, Yung V, Medina-Vogel G. Bat-borne rabies in Latin America. Revista do Instituto de Medicina Tropical de São Paulo. 2015;**57**(1):63-72. DOI: 10.1590/S0036-46652015000100009

[31] WHO, 2017. Available online:http://www.who.int/en/news-room/

fact-sheets/detail/hepatitis-e (Accessed on 10 December 2018)

[32] Rowe IA. Lessons from epidemiology: The burden of liver disease. Digestive Diseases. 2017;**35**(4):304-309. DOI: 10.1159/000456580

[33] Meng XJ, Wiseman B, Elvinger F, Guenette DK, Toth TE, Engle RE, et al. Prevalence of antibodies to hepatitis E virus in veterinarians working with swine and in normal blood donors in the United States and other countries. Journal of Clinical Microbiology. 2002;**40**(1):117-122

[34] Farshadpour F, Taherkhani S, Taherkhani R. Hepatitis E virus infection during pregnancy: The overlooked cause of maternal and fetal mortality. Infectious Disorders Drug Targets. 2018; In press. DOI: 10.2174/1871526518666180530075523

[35] Balayan MS, Andjaparidze AG, Savinskaya SS, Ketiladze ES, Braginsky DM, Savinov AP, et al. Evidence for a virus in non-a, non-B hepatitis transmitted via the fecal-oral route. Intervirology. 1983;**20**(1):23-31

[36] Renou C, Lafeuillade A, Cadranel JF, Pavio N, Pariente A, Allègre T, et al. E virus in HIV-infected patients. AIDS. 2010;**24**(10):1493-1499. DOI: 10.1097/QAD.0b013e32833a29ab

[37] Lee GH, Tan BH, Teo EC, Lim SG, Dan YY, Wee A, et al. Chronic infection with Camelid Hepatitis E virus in a liver transplant recipient who regularly consumes camel meat and Milk. Gastroenterology. 2016;**150**(2):355, e3-357. DOI: 10.1053/j.gastro.2015.10.048

[38] Kamar N, Izopet J, Pavio N, Aggarwal R, Labrique A, Wedemeyer H, et al. Hepatitis E virus infection. Nature Reviews. Disease Primers. 2017;**3**:17086. DOI: 10.1038/nrdp.2017.86

[39] Zhou S, Ren L, Xia X, Miao Z, Huang F, Li Y, et al. Hepatitis E virus infection in HIV-infected patients: A large cohort study in Yunnan province, China. Journal of Medical Virology. 2018;**90**(6):1121-1127. DOI: 10.1002/jmv.25060

[40] Christensen PB, Engle RE, Hjort C, Homburg KM, Vach W, Georgsen J, et al. Time trend of the prevalence of hepatitis E antibodies among farmers and blood donors: A potential zoonosis in Denmark. Clinical Infectious Diseases. 2008;**47**(8):1026-1031. DOI: 10.1086/591970

[41] Mansuy JM, Legrand-Abravanel F, Calot JP, Peron JM, Alric L, Agudo S, et al. High prevalence of anti-hepatitis E virus antibodies in blood donors from south West France. Journal of Medical Virology. 2008;**80**(2):289-293

[42] Lucarelli C, Spada E, Taliani G, Chionne P, Madonna E, Marcantonio C, et al. High prevalence of anti-hepatitis E virus antibodies among blood donors in Central Italy, February to march 2014. Euro Surveillance. 2016;**21**(30). DOI: 10.2807/1560-7917.ES.2016.21.30.30299

[43] Aydin H, Uyanik MH, Karamese M, Timurkan MO. Seroprevalence of Hepatitis E Virus in humans working with animals in non-porcine consumption areas of Turkey. Poster P-1425 presented in 26th European Congress of Clinical Microbiology and Infectious Diseases, 09-12 April 2016, Amsterdam, Netherlands

[44] Bura M, Bukowska A, Bura A, Michalak M, Mozer-Lisewska I. Hepatitis E virus antibodies in HIV-infected patients and blood donors from western Poland: A preliminary report. Advances in Clinical and Experimental Medicine. 2017;**26**(4):577-579. DOI: 10.17219/acem/62353

[45] Zeng H, Wang L, Liu P, Liao L, Wang L, Shao Y. Seroprevalence

of hepatitis E virus in HIV-infected patients in China. AIDS. 2017;**31**(14):2019-2021. DOI: 10.1097/QAD.0000000000001585

[46] Andersson MI, Stead PA, Maponga T, van der Plas H, Preiser W. Hepatitis E virus infection: An underdiagnosed infection in transplant patients in southern Africa? Journal of Clinical Virology. 2015;**70**:23-25. DOI: 10.1016/j.jcv.2015.06.081

[47] Schulz M, Beha D, Plehm K, Zöllner C, Hofmann J, Schott E. High prevalence of anti-hepatitis E virus antibodies in outpatients with chronic liver disease in a university medical center in Germany. European Journal of Gastroenterology & Hepatology. 2016;**28**(12):1431-1436

[48] Abravanel F, Lhomme S, Fougère M, Saune K, Alvarez M, Péron JM, et al. HEV infection in French HIV-infected patients. The Journal of Infection. 2017;**74**(3):310-313. DOI: 10.1016/j.jinf.2016.12.004

[49] Farshadpour F, Taherkhani S, Taherkhani R. Hepatitis E virus infection during pregnancy: The overlooked cause of maternal and fetal mortality. Infectious Disorders Drug Targets. 2018, . In press. DOI: 10.2174/1871526518666180530075523

[50] Khuroo MS, Khuroo MS, Khuroo NS. Hepatitis E: Discovery, global impact, control and cure. World Journal of Gastroenterology. 2016;**22**(31):7030-7045. DOI: 10.3748/wjg.v22.i31.7030

[51] Panda SK, Thakral D, Rehman S. Hepatitis E virus. Reviews in Medical Virology. 2007;**17**(3):151-180

[52] Roque-Afonso AM, Pavio N. Foodborne transmission of hepatitis E virus from raw pork liver sausage, France. Emerging Infectious Diseases. 2014;**20**(11):1945-1947. DOI: 10.3201/eid2011.140791

[53] Smith DB, Simmonds P, International Committee on Taxonomy of Viruses Hepeviridae Study Group, Jameel S, Emerson SU, Harrison TJ, et al. Consensus proposals for classification of the family Hepeviridae. The Journal of General Virology. 2014;**95**(Pt 10):2223-2232

[54] Pavio N, Doceul V, Bagdassarian E, Johne R. Recent knowledge on hepatitis E virus in Suidae reservoirs and transmission routes to human. Veterinary Research. 2017;**48**(1):78. DOI: 10.1186/s13567-017-0483-9

[55] Drexler JF, Seelen A, Corman VM, Fumie Tateno A, Cottontail V, Melim Zerbinati R, et al. Bats worldwide carry hepatitis E virus-related viruses that form a putative novel genus within the family Hepeviridae. Journal of Virology. 2012;**86**(17):9134-9147. DOI: 10.1128/JVI.00800-12

[56] Han HJ, Wen HL, Zhou CM, Chen FF, Luo LM, Liu JW, et al. Bats as reservoirs of severe emerging infectious diseases. Virus Research. 2015;**205**:1-6. DOI: 10.1016/j.virusres.2015.05.006

[57] Shrestha MP, Scott RM, Joshi DM, Mammen MP Jr, Thapa GB, Thapa N, et al. Safety and efficacy of a recombinant hepatitis E vaccine. The New England Journal of Medicine. 2007;**356**(9):895-903

[58] Zhu FC, Zhang J, Zhang XF, Zhou C, Wang ZZ, Huang SJ, et al. Efficacy and safety of a recombinant hepatitis E vaccine in healthy adults: A large-scale, randomised, double-blind placebo-controlled, phase 3 trial. Lancet. 2010;**376**(9744):895-902. DOI: 10.1016/S0140-6736(10)61030-6

[59] Zhang J, Zhang XF, Huang SJ, Wu T, Hu YM, Wang ZZ, et al. Long-term efficacy of a hepatitis E vaccine. The New England Journal of Medicine. 2015;**372**(10):914-922. DOI: 10.1056/NEJMoa1406011

[60] Galvez-Romero G, Salas-Rojas M, Pompa-Mera EN, Chávez-Rueda K, Aguilar-Setién Á. Addition of C3d-P28 adjuvant to a rabies DNA vaccine encoding the G5 linear epitope enhances the humoral immune response and confers protection. Vaccine. 2018;**36**(2):292-298. DOI: 10.1016/j.vaccine.2017.11.047

[61] Deshmukh TM, Lole KS, Tripathy AS, Arankalle VA. Immunogenicity of candidate hepatitis E virus DNA vaccine expressing complete and truncated ORF2 in mice. Vaccine. 2007;**25**(22):4350-4360

[62] Renoux VM, Fleury MJ, Bousarghin L, Gaitan J, Sizaret PY, Touzé A, et al. Induction of antibody response against hepatitis E virus (HEV) with recombinant human papillomavirus pseudoviruses expressing truncated HEV capsid proteins in mice. Vaccine. 2008;**26**(51):6602-6607. DOI: 10.1016/j.vaccine.2008.09.035

[63] Arankalle VA, Lole KS, Deshmukh TM, Srivastava S, Shaligram US. Challenge studies in rhesus monkeys immunized with candidate hepatitis E vaccines: DNA, DNA-prime-protein-boost and DNA-protein encapsulated in liposomes. Vaccine. 2009;**27**(7):1032-1039. DOI: 10.1016/j.vaccine.2008.11.097

[64] Huang WJ, Zhang HY, Harrison TJ, Lan HY, Huang GY, Wang YC. Immunogenicity and protective efficacy in rhesus monkeys of a recombinant ORF2 protein from hepatitis E virus genotype 4. Archives of Virology. 2009;**154**(3):481-488. DOI: 10.1007/s00705-009-0335-7

[65] Gilbert A, Johnson S, Walker N, Wickham C, Beath A, VerCauteren K. Efficacy of Ontario rabies vaccine baits (ONRAB) against rabies infection in raccoons. Vaccine. 2018;**36**(32 Pt B):4919-4926. DOI: 10.1016/j.vaccine.2018.06.052

[66] Dick GW, Kitchen SF, Haddow AJ. Zika virus. I. Isolations and serological specificity. Transactions of the Royal Society of Tropical Medicine and Hygiene. 1952;**46**(5):509-520

[67] World Health Organization (WHO) (2016) Report Zika Situation Neurological Syndrome and Congenital Anomalies. Available from: http://www.who.int/emergencies/zika-virus/situation-report/5-february-2016/en/

[68] Vorou R. Zika virus, vectors, reservoirs, amplifying hosts, and their potential to spread worldwide: What we know and what we should investigate urgently. International Journal of Infectious Diseases. 2016;**48**:85-90. DOI: 10.1016/j.ijid.2016.05.014

[69] Shepherd RC, Williams MC. Studies on viruses in east African bats (Chiroptera). 1. Haemagglutination inhibition and circulation of arboviruses. Zoonoses Research. 1964;**3**(3):125-139

[70] Simpson DI, Williams MC, O'Sullivan JP, Cunningham JC, Mutere FA. Studies on arboviruses and bats (Chiroptera) in East Africa. II. Isolation and haemagglutination-inhibition studies on bats collected in Kenya and throughout Uganda. Annals of Tropical Medicine and Parasitology. 1968;**62**(4):432-440

[71] Calisher CH, Childs JE, Field HE, Holmes KV, Schountz T. Bats: Important reservoir hosts of emerging viruses. Clinical Microbiology Reviews. 2006;**19**(3):531-545

[72] Bittar C, Machado RRG, Comelis MT, Bueno LM, Morielle-Versute E, Beguelini MR, et al. Lack of serological and molecular evidence of arbovirus infections in bats from Brazil. PLoS One. 2018;**13**(11):e0207010. DOI: 10.1371/journal.pone.0207010

[73] Garg H, Mehmetoglu-Gurbuz T, Joshi A. Recent advances in Zika virus vaccines. Viruses. 2018;**10**(11):E631. DOI: 10.3390/v10110631

[74] Beck C, Jimenez-Clavero MA, Leblond A, Durand B, Nowotny N, Leparc-Goffart I, et al. Flaviviruses in Europe: Complex circulation patterns and their consequences for the diagnosis and control of West Nile disease. International Journal of Environmental Research and Public Health. 2013;**10**(11):6049-6083. DOI: 10.3390/ijerph10116049

[75] Rewar S, Mirdha D. Transmission of Ebola virus disease: An overview. Annals of Global Health. 2014;**80**(6):444-451. DOI: 10.1016/j.aogh.2015.02.005

[76] Zhou P, Chionh YT, Irac SE, Ahn M, Jia Ng JH, Fossum E, et al. Unlocking bat immunology: Establishment of *Pteropus alecto* bone marrow-derived dendritic cells and macrophages. Scientific Reports. 2016;**6**:38597. DOI: 10.1038/srep38597

[77] Marzi A, Mire CE. Current Ebola virus vaccine progress. BioDrugs. 2019. In press. DOI: 10.1007/s40259-018-0329-7

[78] Banerjee A, Kulcsar K, Misra V, Frieman M, Mossman K. Bats and coronaviruses. Viruses. 2019;**11**(1):E41. DOI: 10.3390/v11010041

[79] Shi Z, Hu Z. A review of studies on animal reservoirs of the SARS coronavirus. Virus Research. 2008;**33**(1):74-87. DOI: 10.1016/j.virusres.2007.03.012

Section 5

GMO-based Vaccines and their Regulatory Affairs

Chapter 5

GMO Regulatory Aspects of Novel Investigational Vaccine Candidates

Amaya Leunda and Katia Pauwels

Abstract

Recent scientific and technical developments create novel opportunities for vaccine development. Regulatory compliance has to be ensured from preclinical research to market authorization, whereby different legal frameworks that go beyond quality, efficacy or patient safety aspects need to be taken into account. As academia and start-ups are often focused on gathering scientific evidence, the regulatory maze is often regarded by applicants as challenging in the overall pathway to clinical translation. This is particularly true for applications concerning vaccine candidates containing or consisting of genetically modified organisms (GMOs). Active communication between applicants and competent authorities or advisory bodies early in the development stages facilitates a correct implementation of the regulatory frameworks and is of utmost importance to identify challenges or hurdles in order to avoid unnecessary delay in scientific review. Based on the state-of-play in Belgium, this chapter discusses examples of regulatory journeys of applications with genetically modified viral vectors and novel vaccine candidates that have been reviewed by GMO national competent authorities in Belgium and in Europe. They highlight the need of having a comprehensive view of global perspectives early in the development to facilitate the translation of research to clinical development or even market authorization.

Keywords: novel vaccine candidates, GMO, European directives, regulatory challenges, environmental risk assessment

1. Introduction

Recent progress in disease comprehension combined with new technology performances creates novel opportunities for vaccine development in various health sectors. The last decade has seen a significant increase in the development of prophylactic medicines aiming at preventing infectious diseases or immunotherapeutic products to fight non-infectious diseases such as cancers. Both biopharmaceuticals are regarded as vaccines because they elicit an immune response, either against a pathogenic microorganism or against the host's own tumour cells. Among these investigational medicinal products (IMP) for human use currently studied in clinical trials (CT), various candidate vaccines contain or consist of genetically modified organisms (GMOs). For the purpose of this chapter, this subset of IMPs will be further referred to as GMO vaccine candidates.

As for any medicinal product, the clinical translation of research data is subject to a stringent regulatory framework, with procedures to ensure the quality, safety and efficacy of the product in humans. To conduct a new CT in one country of the

IntechOpen

European Union (EU), a clinical trial authorization must be obtained from the national competent authority, and the CT must be approved by an ethics committee. In the case of a CT involving a GMO vaccine candidate or any IMP containing or consisting of a GMO, an authorization should also be compliant with the provisions of the legislation regarding the use of GMOs.

With the increasing number of authorization requests for CT with a GMO vaccine candidate and the new techniques that emerge for the construction of GMOs, the applicants, the national competent authorities and the different advisory bodies are facing some hurdles that may hamper the initiatives undertaken in the clinical translation of vaccine development in Europe. A first challenge originates from the several legislations with which the conduct of a CT with a GMO should comply in the country where the CT is planned. Different legislations are often under the control of different institutional bodies that may not necessarily interrelate and that may not be easily identified by applicants (see the example of Belgium in **Figure 1**). To a lesser extent, the obligation to follow distinct procedural regulations and the subsequent administrative burden may be a deterrent for them. Similarly, the applicant who plans to undertake a CT with a GMO vaccine candidate in multiple member states of the EU can be confronted with an equal number of country-specific procedures. Indeed, contrary to the standard CTA and ethics committee approval procedures for a CT, national GMO regulatory frameworks are not fully harmonized across the EU, and procedures for application may differ from one country to another. Finally, along with the emergence of new techniques intended for genetic modification, both applicants and authorities or advisory bodies are confronted with an increasing number of questions with respect to the interpretation of the definition of a GMO as laid down in the European GMO legislation.

These challenges have the merit of prompting the debate between the different actors and to initiate exchanges at national and European level with the aim to foster a continued dynamic in innovative research, while ensuring the safety of human health and environment. By means of several examples, this book chapter illustrates several aspects of the implementation of the GMO legislation that are of

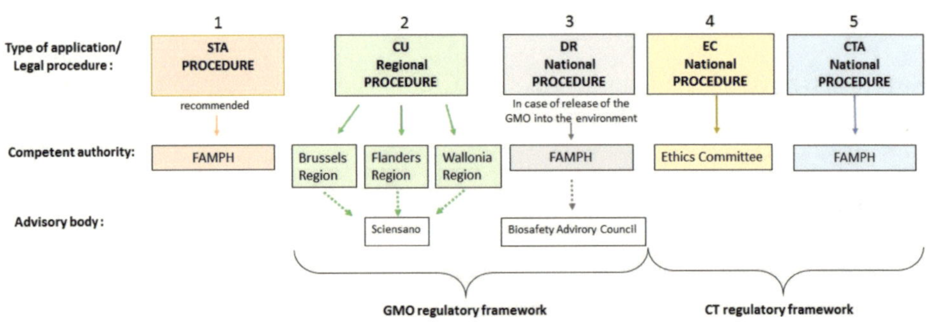

Figure 1.
Overview of Belgian regulatory framework for clinical trials involving an investigational medicinal product containing or consisting of GMOs. STA, scientific and technical advice; FAMHP, Federal Agency of Medicines and Health Products; CU, contained use; DR, deliberate release; EC, Ethics Committee; CTA, clinical trial application. (1) The FAMHP offers to the applicant the possibility to request a STA prior to other mandatory procedures. The STA provides clarity on the GMO status of the IMP involved and the mandatory procedures to follow. (2) The CU procedure is applied to activities with the GMO vaccine candidate taking place in a 'contained' facility. The regional authorities and Sciensano as the advisory body are involved in the CU procedure. The CU procedure and approval are independent of those also associated to a clinical trial. (3) The DR procedure is required when there is a probability of possible release of the GMO into the environment during the clinical trial. An application is submitted to the competent authority, the FAMHP. The application is evaluated by the advisory body (Biosafety Advisory Council) which transmits its advice to the FAMHP. An application under DR framework does not exempt an application under the CU procedure. (4 and 5) Following the national law of 7 May 2004 related to experiments on human, a clinical trial cannot start without a positive advice of the (leading) ethics committee and competent authority.

relevance to CTs with a GMO vaccine candidate. The current state of discussions, an analysis of some of the hurdles that may hamper a smooth clinical translation as well as different options that are available to applicants are reviewed with respect to the Belgian and European regulatory frameworks.

2. Regulatory requirements for GMOs

2.1 The European regulatory framework

The European legislation on GMOs consists of two main Directives covering the use of genetically modified microorganisms (GMMs) in a contained facility (Directive 2009/41/EC) [1] and the deliberate release of GMOs into the environment (Directive 2001/18/EC) [2]. These Directives are mainly aimed at protecting the general population and the environment from potential risks arising from the use of GMMs and GMOs.

According to these Directives GMOs and GMMs are defined as organisms, with the exception of human beings, in which the genetic material has been altered in a way that does not occur naturally by mating and/or natural recombination. The definition of a GMO is both technology and process oriented: an organism will fall under the scope of the GMO regulations if it has been developed with the use of certain techniques. Therefore the EU Directives include annexes supplying information regarding the techniques that result in genetic modification, those that are not considered to result in genetic modification or those that result in genetic modification but yield organisms that are excluded from the scope of the directives (**Table 1**).

The GMO aspects of clinical trials with medicinal products containing or consisting of GMOs, including GMO vaccine candidates, are governed by national procedures implementing the GMO Directives. However, not all member states have the same approach in implementing provisions relating to deliberate release (DR) into the environment (Directive 2001/18/EC) and/or contained use (CU) (Directive 2009/41/EC) in the specific case of clinical trials. A first report on the approaches adopted by several member states in this matter has been commissioned by the European Commission (EC) and dates back to 2007 [3]. In 2018, recognizing the developments in novel medicinal products and the need of applicants of investigational products to have an up-to-date overview of regulatory requirements, a repository of national requirements was created [4]. The approaches adopted by Bulgaria, Germany, Hungary, Ireland, Slovakia, Slovenia, Spain, Sweden and the Netherlands on the one hand, and those prevailing in Denmark on the other, illustrate two extremes. In the first mentioned member states, only the "Deliberate Release' framework is used to assess and manage the risks for human health and the environment, while in Denmark the biological confinement of medicinal products containing or consisting of GMOs and their use in controlled hospital environments trigger the application of the 'Contained Use' regulatory framework only.

One of the important differences between Directive 2009/41/EC and Directive 2001/18/EC is that the latter requests the applicant to submit an environmental risk assessment (ERA). An ERA implies an assessment of the environmental impact of the GMO with regard to the potential risks for human health and the environment. Purely medical aspects concerning the efficacy of the IMP and its safety for the treated patient, as well as aspects related to social, economic or ethical considerations, are outside the scope of the ERA report. The ERA methodology for GMOs developed over the past decades is largely harmonized in many legislative systems and comprises the following steps: (1) hazard identification, (2) hazard characterization, (3) assessment of likelihood, (4) risk estimation and (5) evaluation of

Directive 2009/41/EC	Directive 2001/18/EC
Article 2 (a) 'micro-organism' means any microbiological entity, cellular or non-cellular, capable of replication or of transferring genetic material, including viruses, viroids, animal and plant cells in culture; (b) 'genetically modified micro-organism' (GMM) shall mean a micro-organism in which the genetic material has been altered in a way that does not occur naturally by mating and/or natural recombination. Within the terms of this definition: (i) genetic modification occurs at least through the use of the techniques listed in Annex I, Part A; (ii) the techniques listed in Annex I, Part B, are not considered to result in genetic modification; **Article 3** [...] this Directive shall not apply: - where genetic modification is obtained through the use of the techniques/methods listed in Annex II, Part A	**Article 2** (1) 'organism' means any biological entity capable of replication or of transferring genetic material; (2) 'genetically modified organism (GMO)' means an organism, with the exception of human beings, in which the genetic material has been altered in a way that does not occur naturally by mating and/or natural recombination; Within the terms of this definition: (a) genetic modification occurs at least through the use of the techniques listed in Annex I A, Part 1; (b) the techniques listed in Annex I A, Part 2, are not considered to result in genetic modification. **Article 3.1** This Directive shall not apply to organisms obtained through the techniques of genetic modification listed in Annex I B.
Annex I **Part A** Techniques of genetic modification referred to in Article 2(b)(i) are, *inter alia*: (1) Recombinant nucleic acid techniques involving the formation of new combinations of genetic material by the insertion of nucleic acid molecules produced by whatever means outside an organism, into any virus, bacterial plasmid or other vector system and their incorporation into a host organism in which they do not naturally occur but in which they are capable of continued propagation. (2) Techniques involving the direct introduction into a micro-organism of heritable material prepared outside the micro-organism including micro-injection, macro-injection and micro-encapsulation. (3) Cell fusion or hybridisation techniques where live cells with new combinations of heritable genetic material are formed through the fusion of two or more cells by means of methods that do not occur naturally.	**Annex I A** **Techniques referred to in Article 2(2)** **Part 1** Techniques of genetic modification referred to in Article 2(2)(a) are *inter alia*: (1) Recombinant nucleic acid techniques involving the formation of new combinations of genetic material by the insertion of nucleic acid molecules produced by whatever means outside an organism, into any virus, bacterial plasmid or other vector system and their incorporation into a host organism in which they do not naturally occur but in which they are capable of continued propagation; (2) Techniques involving the direct introduction into an organism of heritable material prepared outside the organism including micro-injection, macro-injection and micro-encapsulation; (3) Cell fusion (including protoplast fusion) or hybridisation techniques where live cells with new combinations of heritable genetic material are formed through the fusion of two or more cells by means of methods that do not occur naturally.
Annex I **Part B** Techniques referred to in Article 2(b)(ii) which are not considered to result in genetic modification, on condition that they do not involve the use of recombinant-nucleic acid molecules or GMMs made by techniques/ methods other than techniques/methods excluded by Annex II, Part A: (1) *in vitro* fertilisation; (2) natural processes such as: conjugation, transduction, transformation; (3) polyploidy induction.	**Annex I A** **Techniques referred to in Article 2(2)** **Part 2** Techniques referred to in Article 2(2)(b) which are not considered to result in genetic modification, on condition that they do not involve the use of recombinant nucleic acid molecules or genetically modified organisms made by techniques/methods other than those excluded by Annex IB: (1) *in vitro* fertilisation, (2) natural processes such as: conjugation, transduction, transformation, (3) polyploidy induction.

Directive 2009/41/EC	Directive 2001/18/EC
Annex II **Part A** Techniques or methods of genetic modification yielding micro-organisms to be excluded from the Directive on the condition that they do not involve the use of recombinant-nucleic acid molecules or GMMs other than those produced by one or more of the techniques/methods listed below: (1) Mutagenesis. (2) Cell fusion (including protoplast fusion) of prokaryotic species that exchange genetic material by known physiological processes. (3) Cell fusion (including protoplast fusion) of cells of any eukaryotic species, including production of hybridomas and plant cell fusions. (4) Self-cloning consisting in the removal of nucleic acid sequences from a cell of an organism which may or may not be followed by reinsertion of all or part of that nucleic acid (or a synthetic equivalent) with or without prior enzymic or mechanical steps, into cells of the same species or into cells of phylogenetically closely related species which can exchange genetic material by natural physiological processes where the resulting micro-organism is unlikely to cause disease to humans, animals or plants. Self-cloning may include the use of recombinant vectors with an extended history of safe use in the particular micro-organisms.	**Annex I B** **Techniques referred to in Article 3** Techniques/methods of genetic modification yielding organisms to be excluded from the Directive, on the condition that they do not involve the use of recombinant nucleic acid molecules or genetically modified organisms other than those produced by one or more of the techniques/methods listed below are: (1) mutagenesis, (2) cell fusion (including protoplast fusion) of plant cells of organisms which can exchange genetic material through traditional breeding methods.

Modified from [31].

Table 1.
The definition of a GMO according to the EU directives [1, 2].

risk management options followed by (6) a conclusion on the acceptability (or not) of the overall impact of the use of the GMO on human health and the environment, taking into account the management strategies applied. Another feature of Directive 2001/18/EC is the mandatory public consultation.

In the context of a marketing authorization application (MAA), it is important to note that Regulation (EC) No 726/2004 [5] laying down procedures for authorization and supervision of medicinal products requests an ERA similar to the ERA applied under Directive 2001/18/EC for medicinal products containing or consisting of GMOs. In practice, the scientific evaluation of the GMO, like any other MAA, is performed through a centralized authorization procedure across the EU. During this process, the European Medicines Agency holds consultations with the competent authorities (CA) of each member states established under Directive 2001/18/EC with respect to the evaluation of the environmental risk aspects. Therefore, even though a contained use-only procedure may have been accepted for a CT involving a GMO, an ERA will need to be submitted according to the provisions of Regulation (EC) 726/2004 should the IMP reach MAA.

2.2 State of the art in Belgium

In Europe, Belgium is one of the most active countries in terms of CTs undertaken with GMO vaccine candidates [6]. This is also observed by the total number of requests submitted to the Belgian authorities for new CTs involving an IMP containing or consisting of a GMO from 2009 to 2018 (**Figure 2**). Until 2018, the number of requests registered annually remained relatively stable, after which a marked increase was observed. These applications involve CT with IMP containing or consisting of a

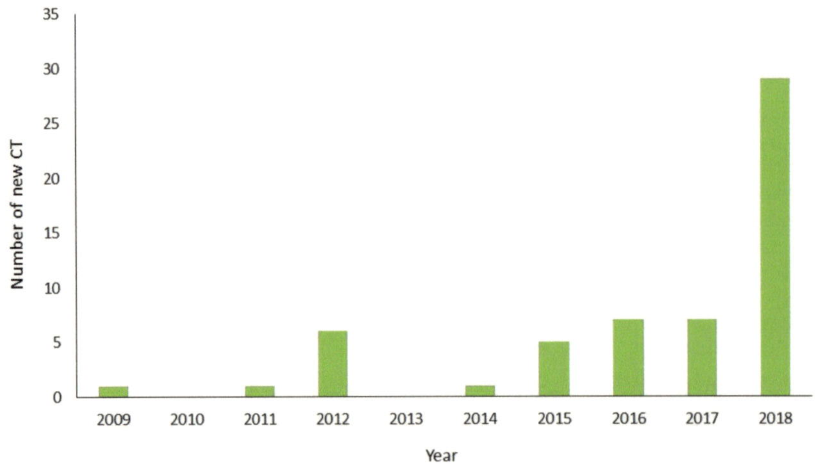

Figure 2.
Number of new clinical trials involving an investigational medicinal product containing or consisting of GMOs since 2009 to 2018 in Belgium. A new clinical trial with a GMO can take place in different clinical centres at the same time. The investigational medicinal product can be directed against infectious, cardiovascular, autoimmune or hereditary diseases but also gastrointestinal disorders, inflammation or cancer.

GMO developed against infectious diseases or cancer, as well as CT with GMOs aiming to treat cardiovascular, autoimmune or hereditary diseases, gastrointestinal disorder or inflammation. Among all these IMPs, around 70% consist of GMO vaccine candidates for prophylactic or therapeutic purposes (data not showed).

GMO vaccine candidates are mainly composed of viral vectors containing one or more specific genetic sequences whose expression in the human body will enhance the immune response against an infectious agent or tumour cells (**Figure 3**). Recently, an increasing number of clinical studies have been realized using autologous or allogenic immune cells that have been genetically modified *ex vivo* in order to express specific receptors able to recognize tumour cells when infused back into the patient body [7]. A minor part of the GMO vaccine candidates consists of the targeted infectious microorganism which is genetically modified *in vitro* to become attenuated yet still capable to trigger an immune response.

In Belgium a clinical trial with an IMP containing or consisting of a GMO can fall into the framework of the CU only or the CU and DR legislations. The GMO procedural pathway is chosen and applied on a case-by-case basis in order to guarantee proportionate and scientifically robust evaluations. To aid in the determination of the legal procedure(s), the applicant is invited to evaluate if at any stage of the CT, the general population and the environment can be exposed to the IMP.

In case physical barriers, or a combination of physical barriers together with chemical and/or biological barriers, are used to limit the contact with the general population and the environment, the CT and related activities have to comply with the Belgian legislation on CU of GMOs. Generally, activities such as the preparation, administration or storage of the IMP should follow the CU procedure only.

In general, a CU procedure suffices when there is no possible release of the GMO in the environment (e.g. the GMO is administered in clinical centres only, and there is no spreading of the GMO when subjects leave the centre) or if proper management procedures and/or working practices are implemented to prevent such a release. On the contrary, when there is a probability of release into the environment (e.g. the subject leaves the clinical centre, and close contacts of the subject may become exposed to the GMO) which cannot be avoided by proper management procedures or working practices, a notification according to the DR procedure

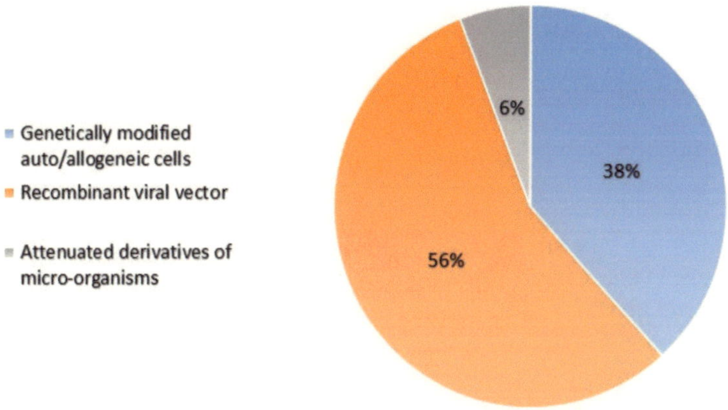

Figure 3.
Types of GMOs used as investigational medicinal products in clinical trials carried out in Belgian clinical centres and corresponding percentage of the total requests from 2009 to 2018. Globally, three main types of GMOs are used: autologous or allogeneic human cells that have been genetically modified ex vivo and reintroduced in a human body (blue), viral vectors genetically modified to carry the gene sequence of interest (orange) and attenuated derivatives of microorganisms that can operate as vaccines (grey).

will additionally be required, and an ERA should be performed. Considerations that are taken into account to determine if a DR notification is needed are the probability of shedding of the GMO, hazards associated to the shedding should it occur, probability of spreading, or whether the GMO is also taken (administered) at home. Procedures for clinical trials within the DR framework are perceived as more cumbersome than those under CU, both for the applicants and for the governmental institutions that are reviewing the applications.

3. New technologies for vaccine development facing regulatory frameworks

For many human infectious diseases no satisfactory vaccine is currently available. Hence, public health needs are continuous incentives for further research and development. Scientific advances not only contributed to the development of novel vaccines that trigger the immune system for prophylactic purposes against infectious diseases but also offered opportunities in gene transfer for (cancer) immunotherapy and the treatment of tumours. Numerous examples have reached clinical development and in some cases even commercialization, even though the interpretation and/or implementation of the regulatory maze is often regarded as challenging by applicants. This section discusses recent developments illustrating the unique features and challenges for GMO vaccines with respect to the current GMO regulation.

3.1 Dengvaxia

Dengvaxia is a GMO vaccine that recently obtained marketing authorization in the EU. This live attenuated vaccine is indicated for the prevention of dengue disease caused by dengue virus serotypes 1, 2, 3 and 4 in individuals living in endemic areas. The vaccine was developed using the attenuated yellow fever vaccine strain as a vector, which has been genetically modified to express the prM and E genes from the four different dengue virus serotypes. The administered vaccine thus contains four different virus constructs, each of which contains the prM and E genes from a different dengue virus serotype. Dengue is by far the most common mosquito-borne viral disease. It is transmitted by Aedes mosquitoes and infects people worldwide (mainly in tropical areas). Tens of millions of cases occur each year resulting in approximately 20,000–25,000 deaths, mainly in children [8]. Because four serologically distinct dengue viruses coexist in dengue-endemic areas, several dengue infections are possible during the patient's lifetime.

The ERA, conducted according to the principles laid down in Directive 2001/18/EC, included among others a consideration of the severity and likelihood of recombination or mutational events that would change the attenuated phenotype of the viral vector to one of virulence. The capacity of the GMO to replicate, disseminate and be transmitted by the Aedes mosquitoes was also evaluated. In addition, both shedding data of subjects receiving the recombinant viruses and the probability of mosquitoes or ticks transmitting the recombinant virus after oral feeding were considered in order to assess the likelihood of dissemination in the human population.

Another aspect that was considered in the context of Directive 2001/18/EC is the detection, traceability and labelling of GMOs. These legal aspects have been further regulated into sectoral legislation for genetically modified food and feed as part of their EU authorization procedure (Regulation EC 1829/2003) [9], and several recommendations have been issued on how analysis methods should be evaluated and validated by the EU Reference Laboratory for Genetically Modified Food and Feed (EURL GMFF). Though Directive 2001/18/EC also covers IMP containing or consisting of GMOs, no sectorial legislation has been developed for IMP. Instead, as Regulation 726/2004, Art 6 (2), refers to Annex IV of Directive 2001/18/EC, traceability must be ensured at all stages of the placing on the market of GMOs (**Table 2**). However, compared to traceability requirements of genetically modified food and feed, it should be noted that much less experience has been gained so far with the validation of methods for the traceability of medicinal GMOs and no such laboratory network has been established to enforce traceability requirements at the European level. During the evaluation of the marketing authorization application of Dengvaxia, it was noticed that traceability methods proposed by the applicant referred to control and monitoring approaches for potentially contaminated effluents at manufacturing sites. However such methods are usually not adapted nor validated for detecting transfer of the donated genetic material to other organisms because the matrix in which the GMOs are supposed to be detected usually differ from those such as effluents of manufacturing sites.

3.2 Plasmid-based live attenuated virus

One of the new avenues to develop novel types of vaccines is the plasmid-based live attenuated virus technology [10]. Upon identification of the protective antigen, this next-generation vaccine platform technology potentially provides for a rapid, versatile and cost-effective vaccine response platform to infectious diseases. The technology circumvents the manufacturing of free live attenuated viral particles as such, which is subject to high-quality control requirements. Instead the genome of an attenuated virus is inserted into human cells by means of a plasmid vector. Human cells that are harbouring the plasmid vector enable the *in vivo* replication of live-attenuated virus (LAV), thereby potentially eliciting immune response and hence immunogenicity. Proof of concept has been delivered for a yellow fever virus strain, and ongoing research will now explore the use of recombinant LAVs as novel vaccines.

The approach of plasmid-based LAV vaccines exemplifies how the pace of innovation and converging technologies may blur current distinctions between a

Regulation (EC) 726/2004	Directive 2001/18/EC
Article 6 (2) In the case of a medicinal product for human use containing or consisting of genetically modified organisms within the meaning of Article 2 of Directive 2001/18/EC, the application shall be accompanied by: (a) a copy of the competent authorities' written consent to the deliberate release into the environment of the genetically modified organisms [...]; (b) the complete technical dossier supplying the information required by Annexes III and IV to Directive 2001/18/EC; (c) the environmental risk assessment in accordance with the principles set out in Annex II to Directive 2001/18/EC; and (d) the results of any investigations performed for the purposes of research or development.	**Annex IV** This Annex describes in general terms the additional information to be provided in the case of notification for placing on the market and information for labelling requirements regarding GMOs: **Part A (7)** Information on the genetic modification for the purposes of placing on one or several registers modifications in organisms, which can be used for the detection and identification of particular GMO products to facilitate post-marketing control and inspection. This information should include where appropriate the lodging of samples of the GMO or its genetic material, with the competent authority and details of nucleotide sequences or other type of information which is necessary to identify the GMO product and its progeny, for example the methodology for detecting and identifying the GMO product, including experimental data demonstrating the specificity of the methodology. Information that cannot be placed, for confidentiality reasons, in the publicly accessible part of the register should be identified.

Table 2.
Legal requirements regarding traceability of an IMP containing or consisting of a GMO in the case of notification for placing on the market.

GMO and a non-GMO, and hence the legal status with regard the legislation on GMOs. Such rapidly evolving fields may also challenge a harmonized understanding of legal definitions across different countries. With respect to GMO regulation, it is not yet clear whether the status of plasmid-based live attenuated viruses will be based on a common interpretation among GMO national competent authorities.

A first element that will contribute to the interpretation can be sought in the GMO status of vaccines that are based on plasmid DNA derived from bacterial cells for use in humans or in animals, the so-called DNA vaccines [11]. Most of the EU member states do not regulate DNA vaccines as a GMO. The reasoning behind this is that a DNA vaccine is not considered an organism. Likewise, human cells transfected with plasmids should not be classified as GMOs, provided that the plasmid is not replicative and is unlikely to integrate into the cell genome. Taking into consideration Article 2 of Directives 2001/18 and 2009/41/EC, and corresponding annexes (**Table 1**), nucleic acid material (DNA or RNA) such as plasmids present under episomal form in a human cell is not considered as heritable material (of the human cell) unless the nucleic acid material is capable of continued propagation, for example, by integration of the nucleic acid material into the genome of the human cell, or when the plasmid contains an origin of eukaryotic replication. It should be noted that the probability of integration cannot be totally excluded for plasmids not known to contain integrative elements or homologous sequences. However, should an integration event occur, the risk for the human population or the environment, associated to the use of transfected human cells, would be negligible. Indeed, human cells can only propagate inside the human body or under controlled *in vitro* conditions. In terms of potential risks for the human population and the environment, it follows that the risk associated to the use of a transfected human cell is negligible provided that the plasmid is not replicative or not integrative.

A second element that prompts reflection on the GMO status, which is of particular relevance for the plasmid-based LAV technology, is associated to plasmids harbouring the full sequence of a virus. In that case the plasmid-transfected human cells may lead to the generation of replication-competent virus particles in the host human cells that eventually can be released into the environment. A plasmid harbouring a virus strain that has been genetically modified would be subjected to the GMO framework. However, the GMO status of plasmids harbouring the full sequence of a naturally occurring virus or attenuated virus has not been determined yet.

3.3 CAR T cells

Therapeutic vaccines for cancer immunotherapy with chimeric antigen receptor (CAR) T cells are another medical development exploiting modern biotechnology tools. Cancer immunotherapy uses the patient's own T cells that have been engineered to express a receptor targeting an antigen on the surface of tumour cells [12–14]. CAR T cell-based immunotherapy has shown remarkable efficacy against human malignancies, thereby providing a promising alternative to allogeneic haematopoietic stem cell transplantation which is known to be associated with severe side effects. It is anticipated that the number of developments using CAR T cells will continue to expand as current research now explores, for example, the potency of (CAR) T cells in solid tumours or the use of allogeneic 'off-the-shelf' T cells. The rapid pace of developments in part has been facilitated by the implementation of gene-editing tools to genetically modify human T cells.

Genome-editing techniques involving the use of site-directed nucleases (SDN), like the ribonucleoprotein-mediated gene editing of cells, make it possible to induce modifications in a predefined region of the genome without the need to introduce foreign (exogenous) DNA [15]. For some applications, the resulting organisms cannot be distinguished from those generated through classic mutagenesis or spontaneous mutations. While addressing how these techniques relate to the European GMO legislation and taking into account that organisms developed through classical mutagenesis are excluded from the EU regulatory framework for GMOs, a number of authorities or advisory bodies of EU members have expressed the opinion that applications of SDN, resulting in small point mutation or indels, could be exempted from the EU GMO regulation on the condition that the nuclease is not stably expressed from a recombinant nucleic acid molecule [16]. Therefore the advent of gene-editing techniques was challenging the boundaries of the GM regulation in the EU, at least until a legal opinion of the Court of Justice of the EU (ECJ) was issued. The ruling declared that organisms produced by mutagenesis techniques, including directed mutagenesis and applications of gene editing, should be regulated under EU GMO law, unless the mutagenesis technique has conventionally been used in a number of applications and has a long safety record [17]. Much opposition has been raised against this ruling, in particular with respect to the inclusion of gene-edited plants within the remit of GMO legislation [18, 19].

The ruling applies to medicinal GMOs as well and will determine the legal status of CAR T cells obtained with gene-editing techniques with respect to GMO legislation. Apart from notifications in the context of CTAs, such an IMP would also require an ERA when reaching MAA (Regulation (EC) 726/2004). However, though human cells may survive in whole blood or synthetic media with a composition similar to human blood, these cells can only propagate inside the human body or under controlled *in vitro* conditions. Human cells will not survive in non-optimized conditions, and it is highly unlikely that the genetic modification of these cells, by means of gene-editing tools, will alter the inherent fitness of human cells for survival in the environment upon their release, much less to cause any adverse effects to human health or animal health. It follows that for MAA involving the use of gene-edited human (autologous) cells, the risks for human health and/or the environment associated to the handling/use of the medical product is negligible.

3.4 Novel oral poliovirus type 2 vaccine candidates

The continuous improvements in DNA synthesis technology also hold promise in the design of new vaccines. Developers may go further than recombinant DNA technology and make a step towards increased rational design, away from existing nucleotide sequences. For example, the genetic code of the virus can be redesigned so that 100% identity is preserved at the protein level with significant differences at the nucleotide level. This codon deoptimization has been described as an approach to generate attenuated viruses that can be used as vaccines [20, 21]. The synthesis of poliovirus (PV) as early as 2002 is considered as one of the first milestones in synthetic genomics [22]. Most recently, a clinical trial has been set-up involving two GMOs consisting of novel live attenuated polio vaccine candidates that have been developed through advanced DNA synthesis technology and codon deoptimization [23]. Though few preliminary questions were related to the GMO status of the novel live attenuated polio vaccines, it was merely the context of the global Polio Eradication Initiative and the associated efforts to minimize poliovirus facility-associated risks, as defined in the WHO's Global Action Plan III (GAP III) [24] that added to the complexity of the legal procedure.

Poliovirus has a particular status from a global world health perspective since the launch of the global Polio Eradication Initiative in 1988. Immunization with trivalent live, attenuated oral poliovirus vaccine (OPV), composed of three strains OPV1, 2 and 3, has led to a drastic decline in the number of polio cases worldwide. However OPV is genetically unstable and can regain neurovirulence, leading to outbreaks of circulating vaccine-derived poliovirus (cVDPV). In a context of PV type 2 eradication worldwide and because the risk associated to the use of OPV2 was outweighing the benefits, it was decided to withdraw the type 2 component from OPV vaccination campaigns and to introduce the inactivated poliovirus vaccine, which is more expensive and relatively more cumbersome to administer. Nevertheless, due to its induced superior mucosal immunity, monovalent OPV2 is still used in responses to outbreaks of cVDPV2, thereby challenging the feasibility of eradication of PV2 [25]. It is within this context that a global consortium of investigators, governmental, non-governmental, academic and global health organizations worked on the development of two novel OPV2 vaccine candidates (nOPV2) with better genetic stability and reduced risk to regain a neurovirulent phenotype.

The first-in-human (FIH) phase 1 study was conducted in Belgium. Although the clinical development of such novel vaccines was considered highly desirable from a world health perspective, the launch of a FIH study was considered under severe scrutiny in order to avoid any risk of introducing VDPV in a country declared polio-free for several years. As shedding of the nOPV2 was anticipated for a mean time of 2 weeks, the consortium decided to conduct the FIH phase 1 study with voluntary participants under full containment during 28 days, with strengthened containment measures. Rather unexpectedly, the study showed that ~50% of the subjects still were shedding after having left the full containment period of 28 days. Post-discharge biorisk management measures were applied to prevent the release of the candidate vaccines in the environment and to avoid contact with immune-compromised individuals.

The WHO's Polio Eradication Department encouraged further progress in the clinical study of the novel OPV vaccines and the consortium applied for a phase

II CT with the nOPV2 vaccine candidates. On the basis of shedding and genetic stability data obtained with the FIH study, and the larger size of cohorts to be involved during the phase II study, the consortium applied for an authorization for deliberate release into the environment of the GMOs. In accordance with the Royal Decree transposing Directive 2001/18/EC into Belgian law, an ERA was submitted [26], a public consultation was organized, and a notification according to the provisions of Council Decision 2002/813/EC [27], the so-called summary notification information format (SNIF), was circulated. This enables an exchange of information between the EU member state and the Commission on the basis of relevant information.

It has been the first example to our knowledge of EU member states commenting on the SNIF. One of the concerns raised by neighbouring countries was the transboundary release of the nOPV2, should the healthy volunteers not stay in Belgium during the period of virus shedding. Those concerns are not only related to GMO regulatory provisions but also to GAP III requirements, which describe a biorisk management system addressing areas associated with the design, operation and management for facilities handling poliovirus facilities [28]. It can be concluded that the regulatory pathway to the setup of the two first CT involving nOPV2 revealed an additional complexity involving increased exchanges both at national and international levels.

4. Engagement with regulatory agencies or advisory bodies

4.1 Importance of networking

Medicines become more and more the result of different and converging technologies. For many human infectious diseases, no satisfactory vaccine is currently available, and the development of vaccines containing or consisting of GMOs is one of the innovative technologies implemented to meet some of the public health needs. Regulators involved in medicinal products for humans, as well as in GMOs, need to anticipate these developments, not only by enforcing safety regulations but also by ensuring the scientific review adheres to the principles of proportionality and case-by-case approach. From the applicants' side, it is recognized that the regulatory pathway for novel technologies is complicated and not always straightforward. Early dialogue between applicants, risk assessors and the regulatory authorities is therefore paramount in addressing challenges with clinical translation of novel GMO vaccines.

The steps that were undertaken towards the approval of early phases of a clinical trial investigating nOPV2 vaccine candidates in a post-OPV2-withdrawal era exemplify the importance of liaising among several regulatory agencies and public health institutions covering (international) public health objectives at national, European and global level. At the time the consortium that worked on the development of the nOPV2 vaccine candidates applied for its second clinical trial, it was still not clear whether the nOPV2 vaccine candidates were to be considered under the scope of GAP III. Because the consortium engaged as early as possible with advisory and/or regulatory institutions, the Belgian authorities were prompted to ask the WHO's Containment Advisory Group to clarify the GAP III status of the nOPV2 vaccine candidates and, if these were to fall under the scope of GAP III, how to interpret or implement the GAP III guidelines in a phase II clinical study. The WHO's Containment Advisory Group concluded that, according to the specific terms of usage proposed in the context of the protocol of the CT, the nOPV2 could be used outside the containment requirements of GAP III. It also requested the addition to the trial protocols of environmental monitoring for polioviruses around the trial sites, as well as monitoring of close and family contacts of trial subjects who continued to shed virus after the end of the trial period [29].

This case exemplifies how different aspects of public health interrelate and contribute to the complexity of the regulatory maze to which applicants may be confronted when submitting clinical trial applications. Both the consortium and Belgian authorities liaised with several regulatory agencies and public health institutions covering different (international) public health objectives in order to ensure that risk management measures were proportional to the risk/safety assessment taking into account the intended use, the receiving environment and the likelihood of exposure.

4.2 Interplay GMO-pharma

A concern of developers that is acknowledged by the European Commission is the lack of harmonization of regulatory procedures of clinical trials with regard to the GMO legislative framework. The approval of clinical trials is within the remit of the member states and the interplay between the CT regulation and the GMO regulation might differ between the member states. This non-harmonized approach among member states, detailed under Section 2 of this chapter, is perceived as ineffective for the conduct of multinational clinical trials and as an impediment to the effective translation of research findings into clinical applications.

Very recently the first steps towards a common procedure for a subset of innovative therapies for human use involving the use of GMOs has been agreed upon among member states [30]. It concerns an application form specifically developed for clinical trials involving the use of human cells transduced with retroviral or lentiviral vector systems. Taking into account that the evaluation of clinical trial with respect to the GMO legislation will remain within the remit of national authorities, this initiative can be seen as a significant step towards enhanced communication among regulators. It is also of high value in light of the upcoming therapeutic strategies based on the genetic modification of T cells that target defined antigens presented by tumour cells and aids the patient's own immune system to combat malignant diseases, the so-called CAR- and TCR-modified T cells.

The European Commission continues to foster exchanges among member states with the aim of developing common application forms, increasing cooperation in the risk assessment of applications and identifying issues and questions with respect to the scope of the GMO regulatory framework.

4.3 Scientific and technical advice

As already mentioned, at the time of planning a CT with a GMO in a European member state, the applicant may be confronted to a complex regulatory procedure, exceeding what is required for a standard study with an IMP. Alongside the standard Clinical Trial Application (CTA) and obtaining the advice from the ethics committee, questions regarding the GMO status of the IMP and the proper mandatory procedural steps may arise. In addition, should the IMP be identified as a GMO, the developer will need to identify a distinct competent authority in charge of reviewing the application according to the adequate procedural steps.

As outlined earlier, the determination of the GMO procedural pathway for a CT in Belgium (meaning whether the CU only or both CU and DR procedures must be followed) is subject to a case-by-case examination taking into account the possible release of the GMO into the environment and the possible associated risks. To help the applicant, the competent authority for CTAs offers the possibility to request a scientific and technical advice (STA) prior to the CTA. The main objective of the STA is to facilitate the development of vaccines and therapeutic products by centralizing and analysing the applicant's concerns at the time of starting the CT.

Within the STA, the applicant is invited to request clarifications on the GMO status of the IMP, and on the GMO procedures to be followed, should it decide to proceed with the application. The competent authority for CTAs coordinates the contacts with experts, centralizes their responses and delivers a formal advice to the developer. As such, the STA is a means for developers to engage with the competent authorities and advisory bodies early in the process in order to (i) provide information that would facilitate further process and (ii) avoid possible misunderstandings with regard the GMO status and procedures, which consequently may save time for the developer.

5. Discussion and conclusions

With novel technologies poised to result in the development of novel IMPs and the overall drive for sustained innovation, a number of regulatory hurdles can be identified, which developers face during the development of GMO vaccines. First, EU GMO Directives have been transposed into national legislations that include different regulatory specificities between member states. Second, new technologies may lead to the generation of organisms that are prone to different interpretations with regard to their (GMO) regulatory status, thereby hampering further harmonization of legislations. In addition, aspects such as the relevance of an ERA or detection and traceability requirements become in some cases disproportionate with respect to the actual risks that novel IMP represent for the general population and the environment. Overall, these aspects will increase the need of regulatory agencies and advisory bodies to anticipate the deployment of novel IMP, through continuous engagement with all stakeholders.

The ECJ ruling has initiated the debate concerning the need to rewrite the GMO Directive 2001/18/EC, to have it more fit-for-purpose for the rapid pace of emerging technologies. This is particularly true for gene-editing technologies. Although it is primarily the impact on agri-food applications that has sparked these debates, the ECJ ruling will also have an effect on research and development activities and the development of a category of IMP. It is anticipated that the current debate on the appropriateness of the existing GMO regulatory framework may affect the future regulatory status of GMO medicines. This may have consequences through all stages of development, from R&D, through clinical translation and marketing authorization application.

Aiming to overcome existing hurdles in the regulatory pathway, a number of initiatives have been taken in Belgium and among member states. Key challenges are being addressed, for example, with the STA at Belgian level, and tangible solutions have been formulated, such as the common form for CT with human cells genetically modified *ex vivo* by retro- or lentiviral vectors. It is expected that the need for harmonization and reviewing regulatory frameworks will be the basis of further engagement and exchange between all stakeholders.

New technologies in the field of biotechnology spark promising avenues for the development of novel biopharmaceuticals involving GMOs. Enhanced networking among all stakeholders should be further promoted in order to subject regulatory frameworks to critical review with the aim of keeping them up-to-date with upcoming developments and to support innovation while ensuring quality and safety for patients, the general population and the environment.

Acknowledgements

The authors thank Aline Baldo, Didier Breyer, Fanny Coppens and Nicolas Willemarck (Sciensano) for critical reading. **Figures 2** and **3** result from contributions from Nicolas Willemarck.

Conflict of interest

The authors declare that they have no conflict of interest.

Author details

Amaya Leunda* and Katia Pauwels
Sciensano, Brussels, Belgium

*Address all correspondence to: amaya.leundacasi@sciensano.be

References

[1] Directive 2009/41/EC of the European Parliament and of the Council of 6 May 2009 on the Contained Use of Genetically Modified Micro-Organisms (Recast) [Internet]. Available from: https://eur-lex.europa.eu/legal-content/EN/TXT/PDF/?uri=CELEX:32009L0041&from=EN [Accessed: January 9, 2019]

[2] Directive 2001/18/EC of the European Parliament and of the Council of 12 March 2001 on the Deliberate Release into the Environment of Genetically Modified Organisms and Repealing Council Directive 90/220/EEC [Internet]. Available from: https://eur-lex.europa.eu/resource.html?uri=cellar:303dd4fa-07a8-4d20-86a8-0baaf0518d22.0004.02/DOC_1&format=PDF [Accessed: January 9, 2019]

[3] Analysis of the Applicability of the Contained Use Legislation for Clinical Trials [Internet]. Available from: https://www.genetherapynet.com/download/EU-analysis-Contained-use.pdf [Accessed: January 9, 2019]

[4] Genetically Modified Organism (GMO) Aspects for Investigational Medicinal Products [Internet]. Available from: https://ec.europa.eu/health/human-use/advanced-therapies/gmo_investiganional_en [Accessed: January 9, 2019]

[5] Regulation (EC) No 726/2004 of the European Parliament and of the Council of 31 March 2004 Laying Down Community Procedures for the Authorisation and Supervision of Medicinal Products for Human and Veterinary Use and Establishing a European Medicines Agency [Internet] Available from: https://ec.europa.eu/health/sites/health/files/files/eudralex/vol-1/reg_2004_726/reg_2004_726_en.pdf [Accessed: January 9, 2019]

[6] Florence Kauffmann F, Van Damme P, Leroux-Roels G, Vandermeulen C, Mali S. Clinical trials with GMO-containing vaccines in Europe: Status and regulatory framework. In preparation for submission

[7] Pang Y, Hou X, Yang C, Liu Y, Jiang G. Advances on chimeric antigen receptor-modified T-cell therapy for oncotherapy. Molecular Cancer. 2018;**17**:91. DOI: 10.1186/s12943-018-0840-y

[8] Factsheet about Dengue Fever [Internet] Available from: https://ecdc.europa.eu/en/dengue-fever/facts/factsheet [Accessed: January 9, 2019]

[9] Regulation (EC) No 1829/2003 of the European Parliament and of the Council of 22 September 2003 on Genetically Modified Food and Feed [Internet]. Available from: https://eur-lex.europa.eu/legal-content/EN/TXT/PDF/?uri=CELEX:32003R1829&from=en [Accessed: January 9, 2019]

[10] Plasmid based Live Attenuated Virus [Internet]. Available from: https://rega.kuleuven.be/cmt/jn/viruses/pllav-a-plasmid-based-live-attenuated-vaccine-technology [Accessed: January 9, 2019]

[11] DNA Vaccines [Internet]. Available from: https://www.who.int/biologicals/areas/vaccines/dna/en/ [Accessed: January 9, 2019]

[12] Sharma P, Allison JP. The future of immune checkpoint therapy. Science. 2015;**348**:56-61. DOI: 10.1126/science.aaa8172

[13] Morsut L, Roybal KL, Xiong X, Gordley RM, Coyle SM, Thomson M, et al. Engineering customized cell sensing and response behaviors using synthetic notch receptors. Cell. 2016;**164**:780-791. DOI: 10.1016/j.cell.2016.01.012

[14] June CH, O'Connor RS, Kawalekar O, Ghassemi S, Milone MC. CAR T cell immunotherapy for human cancer. Science. 2018;**359**:1361-1365. DOI: 10.1126/science.aar6711

[15] Pauwels K, Podevin N, Breyer D, Carroll D, Herman P. Engineering nucleases for gene targeting: Safety and regulatory considerations. New Biotechnology. 2014;**31**:18-27. DOI: 10.1016/j.nbt.2013.07.001

[16] Targeted Genome Editing [Internet]. Available from: https://www.biosafety.be/content/targeted-genome-editing [Accessed: January 9, 2019]

[17] Judgment of Court of Justice of the European Union [Internet]. 2018. Available from: https://curia.europa.eu/jcms/upload/docs/application/pdf/2018-07/cp180111en.pdf [Accessed: January 9, 2019]

[18] Casacuberta JM, Puigdomènech P. Proportionate and scientifically sound risk assessment of gene-edited plants. EMBO Reports. 2018;**19**:e46907. DOI: 10.15252/embr.201846907

[19] Statement of the Group of Chief Scientific Advisors : A Scientific Perspective on the Regulatory status of Products Derived from Gene Editing and the Implications for the GMO Directive [Internet]. 2018. Available from: https://ec.europa.eu/info/sites/info/files/2018_11_gcsa_statement_gene_editing_1.pdf [Accessed: January 9, 2019]

[20] Mueller S, Coleman JR, Papamichail D, Ward CB, Nimnual A, Futcher B, et al. Live attenuated influenza virus vaccines by computer-aided rational design. Nature Biotechnology. 2010;**28**:732-736. DOI: 10.1038/nbt.1636

[21] Coleman JR, Papamichail D, Skiena S, Futcher B, Wimmer E, Mueller S. Virus attenuation by genome-scale changes in codon pair bias. Science. 2008;**320**(5884):1784-1787. DOI: 10.1126/science.1155761

[22] Cello J, Paul AV, Wimmer E. Chemical synthesis of poliovirus cDNA: Generation of infectious virus in the absence of natural template. Science. 2002;**297**(5583):1016-1018. DOI: 10.1126/science.1072266

[23] Summary Notification Information Format for the Release of Genetically Modified Organisms Other Than Higher Plants in Accordance with Article 11 of Directive 2001/18/EC [Internet]. Available from: http://gmoinfo.jrc.ec.europa.eu/gmo_report.aspx?CurNot=B/BE/18/BVW2 [Accessed: January 9, 2019]

[24] WHO Global Action Plan to Minimize Poliovirus Facility-Associated Risk After Type-Specific Eradication of Wild Polioviruses and Sequential Cessation of Oral Polio Vaccine Use [Internet]. Available from: http://apps.who.int/iris/bitstream/handle/10665/208872/WHO_POLIO_15.05_eng.pdf [Accessed: January 9, 2019]

[25] Blake IM, Pons-Salort M, Molodecky NA, Diop OM, Chenoweth P, Bandyopadhyay AS, et al. Type 2 poliovirus detection after global withdrawal of trivalent Oral vaccine. The New England Journal of Medicine. 2018;**379**:834-845. DOI: 10.1056/NEJMoa1716677

[26] Advice of the Belgian Biosafety Advisory Council on the Notification B/BE/18/BVW2 of the Centre of the Evaluation of Vaccination [Internet]; University of Antwerp. Available from: https://www.biosafety.be/sites/default/files/bac_2018_0578.pdf [Accessed: January 9, 2019]

[27] Council Decision of 3 October 2002 Establishing, Pursuant to Directive 2001/18/EC of the European Parliament and of the Council, The summary

notification information format for notifications Concerning the Deliberate Release into the Environment of Genetically Modified Organisms for Purposes Other than for Placing on the Market [Internet]. Available from: https://eur-lex.europa.eu/legal-content/EN/TXT/PDF/?uri=CELEX:32002D0813&from=EN [Accessed: January 9, 2019]

[28] Previsani N, Tangermann RH, Tallis G, Jafari HS. World Health Organization guidelines for containment of poliovirus following type-specific polio eradication—Worldwide. Morbidity and Mortality Weekly Report. 2015;**64**:913-917

[29] Report on the Containment Requirements of nOPV2 Vaccine Candidates [Internet]. Available from: http://polioeradication.org/wp-content/uploads/2018/08/containment-advisory-group-teleconference-3-on-noOPV2-S19-Sabin2-novel-strains-7-june-2018-20180814.pdf [Accessed: January 9, 2019]

[30] Major Developments in Advanced T: GMO Requirements for Investigational Products [Internet]. Available from: https://ec.europa.eu/health/human-use/advanced-therapies_en [Accessed: January 9, 2019]

[31] Breyer D, Herman P, Brandenburger A, Gheysen G, Remaut E, Soumillion P, et al. Genetic modification through oligonucleotide-mediated mutagenesis. A GMO regulatory challenge? Environmental Biosafety Research. 2009;**8**:57-64. DOI: 10.1051/ebr/2009007

Section 6

Vaccinia-virus-derived Vectors for Zoonotic Diseases

Chapter 6

Vaccinia Virus-Derived Vectors in Leishmaniases Vaccine Development

Dulcilene Mayrink de Oliveira, Jonatan Marques Campos, Soraia de Oliveira Silva and Maria Norma Melo

Abstract

Due to an increase in the incidence of leishmaniases worldwide, the development of new strategies such as prophylactic vaccines to prevent infection and decrease the diseases has become a high priority. The development of vaccines against the various species of pathogenic *Leishmania* to humans has been hampered, in part, by the inefficient stimulation of the protective cellular immunity promoted by the administration of purified or recombinant antigens, indicating the need for new approaches. Viral vectors represent an attractive way to deliver and present vaccine antigens that may offer advantages over traditional platforms. Among the most attractive and efficient viral vectors in inducing a cellular immune response, vaccinia virus has been the most used in leishmaniases vaccine trials. The first report of the use of recombinant vaccinia virus (VACV) in the induction of protection against *Leishmania* infection was made in 1993. Since then, several *Leishmania* spp. antigenic subunits were cloned into recombinant VACV. Although highly attenuated poxviral vectors are capable of inducing protective immunity against *Leishmania* spp., their limitation in replicative capacity reduces their potential as compared to replicative vectors. In order to achieve a balance between safety and replication, several VACV strains with intermediate phenotype have been developed.

Keywords: leishmaniases, vaccines, viral vectors, recombinant vaccinia virus, VACV

1. Introduction

Leishmaniases are important neglected tropical diseases (NTD) caused by protozoan parasites from the genus *Leishmania* Ross, 1903, of which more than 20 species are pathogenic to humans. Such parasites are transmitted by about 30 species of infected female sandflies (genus *Phlebotomus* and *Lutzomyia)* [1, 2], and their biological cycle alternates between the amastigote forms (obligatory intracellular), in the mammalian host, and promastigote forms (extracellular), in the vector digestive tract [3]. The diseases present a range of mammalian hosts, such as canids, rodents, marsupials, edentates, and primates, both human and nonhuman. The species that infect humans are distributed in two subgenera: *Leishmania* and *Viannia*, based on the development of the parasites inside the insect vector digestive tracts. Depending on the *Leishmania* species and the host's immune status, leishmaniases present a broad spectrum of clinical manifestations, which can be divided into two main groups: (I) visceral leishmaniasis (VL) caused by *Leishmania (Leishmania) infantum* (syn. *L. (L.) chagasi)* and *L. (L.) donovani* and (II) tegumentary leishmaniasis (TL), with cutaneous form (CL) caused by *L. (L.) major*, *L. (L.) amazonensis*, *L. (L.) mexicana*, *L. (L.) aethiopica*, *L. (Viannia) braziliensis*, *L. (V.) guyanensis,* and *L. (V.) panamensis* and the mucocutaneous form (MCL) mainly caused by *L. (V.) braziliensis* and *L. (V.) guyanensis*, in the New World, and *L. (L.) aethiopica,* in the Old World [4, 5].

It is estimated that 14 million people are infected worldwide, and 350 million are at risk of infection. Approximately 1.3 million new cases are registered annually [3]. According to the Global Burden of Disease Study (GDB) 2010, about 50,000 people die each year from the diseases, resulting in 3.3 million disability-adjusted life years (DALY) lost [6]. In recent decades, several *Leishmania* species have spread to non-endemic areas [7].

According to the World Health Organization (WHO), leishmaniases are among the emerging and uncontrolled category 1 diseases, and their prevention is based primarily on three parameters: (I) vector control, (II) control of parasitic reservoir animals, and (III) research and development of new vaccine candidates [8]. Spraying of intra- and peri-domiciliary residual insecticides has been crucial in the control of sandflies. However, there is concern about the emergence of vector resistance to dichlorodiphenyltrichloroethane (DDT), especially in highly endemic areas [9]. The chemotherapeutic treatment of infected dogs, the main reservoirs of the parasite in VL, reduces or eliminates symptoms. Yet, many animals are still able to transmit the parasite, remaining the epidemiological risk. Other measures, such as topical insecticides and impregnated collars, are expensive and difficult to implement in national control programs [10]. In the absence of effective strategies, vaccine development is cost-effective in controlling leishmaniases. It is estimated that a vaccine with a 70% efficacy providing protection for 10 years is able to prevent 41–144 thousand CL cases in seven Latin American countries (Bolivia, Brazil, Colombia, Ecuador, Mexico, Peru, and Venezuela) with an inferior cost than the currently recommended treatments. As for VL, even a vaccine that provides protection for only 5 years with a 50% efficacy would still be more economically feasible compared to current treatments [9].

The first leishmaniases vaccination attempts, named leishmanization, were based on the observation that an individual cured of a cutaneous lesion became refractory to reinfection [7, 8]. In leishmanization, the infectious lesion material, later replaced by the cultured parasites, was used in the inoculation of uninfected individuals. This method was interrupted due to a number of factors, including quality control, persistence of the parasite in the body, the emergence of the HIV virus in the 1980s, and ethical reasons [11].

The first generation of vaccines emerged from leishmanization and comprises heat or phenol-killed promastigote forms associated with different adjuvants, including BCG (*Mycobacterium bovis,* bacillus Calmette-Guérin) and irradiated or attenuated live promastigotes. However, the standardization of vaccines derived from parasites in culture hinders their register by the competent national institutions [7, 8]. Human vaccination using dead strains of *Leishmania* spp. dates back to the late 1930s was a pioneering strategy among Brazilian scientists. Phase III clinical trials conducted in Ecuador and Colombia utilized a Brazilian vaccine called Leishvacin®, composed of *L. amazonensis* killed promastigotes in association with BCG adjuvant, which demonstrated safety but low efficacy [10, 11]. After a period of 4 years of commercial production by Bioquímica do Brasil (BIOBRÁS, Brazil), Leishvacin® is now only produced in a nonindustrial way in research laboratories for clinical assays. The vaccine is also accepted as an immunotherapeutic agent with or without association with Glucantime® (Rhône

Poulenc Rorer, France), for the treatment of resistant individuals or for the ones Glucantime® induces high toxicity. Of late, three forms of vaccines consisting of *L. major*, *L. amazonensis*, and *L. Mexicana* were evaluated by first-generation vaccines of human clinical trials [12].

The second generation of vaccines includes purified or recombinant *Leishmania spp.* proteins [8]. In Brazil, in 2003 and 2006, respectively, two second-generation vaccines against canine visceral leishmaniasis (CVL), Leishmune® (Fort Dodge, Brazil) and Leish-Tec® (Hertape Calier, Brazil), were registered. Leishmune® is composed of a purified fraction of the fucose-mannose ligand (FML) isolated from *L. donovani* promastigotes, associated with the saponin adjuvant. Their formulation has been shown to be safe, protective, and highly immunogenic for dogs, in addition to being able to prevent the transmission of CVL [13]. However, since November 2014, the vaccine has been suspended for manufacturing and marketing due to noncompliance with the complete requirements of the Ministério da Agricultura, Pecuária e Abastecimento (MAPA, Brazil) for phase III studies on vaccine efficacy (NOTA TÉCNICA N° 038/2014/DFIP/DAS). As for Leish-Tec®, it is composed of the *L. donovani* recombinant A2 protein associated with the saponin adjuvant. A2 is a highly expressed surface protein in the amastigote form of *L. donovani* and was the first virulence factor identified in *Leishmania* spp.; such protein is necessary for the survival of the parasite in the mammalian host and is involved in the visceralization of the pathogen during infection [14]. Dogs immunized with Leish-Tec® and experimentally infected by *L. infantum* were able to develop a partially protective immune response against CVL, presenting positive parasitism in the bone marrow 9 months after the challenge [15]. In Europe, the first CVL vaccine registered and commercially available in 2011 was LiESP/QA-21, named CaniLeish® (Virbac, France), a second-generation vaccine composed of *L. infantum* excreted/secreted recombinant proteins (LiESP) associated with a highly purified fraction of *Quillaja saponaria* saponin (QA-21) as an adjuvant [16]. Clinical trials in dogs vaccinated with CaniLeish® and experimentally infected by *L. infantum* demonstrated, after 1 year, reduced parasite load, specific cellular immune response, and decreased chance of relapses [17]. Another vaccine currently commercialized in Europe is LetiFend®, whose active principle is a recombinant chimeric protein, named Protein Q, composed by the fusion of five epitopes of the acidic ribosomal proteins LiP2A, LiP2B, LiP0, and the histone H2A of *L. infantum*. The efficacy of vaccination in a large-scale dog population demonstrated that LetiFend® is a novel, safe, and effective vaccine for the active immunization of noninfected dogs from 6 months of age in reducing the risk of developing clinical visceral leishamaniasis after natural infection with *L. infantum* [18].

Likewise A2, FML, LiESP, and Protein Q, several other *Leishmania*-derived antigens have already been identified as immunogenic based on T cell clones, due to its abundance and specific location in the parasite, by screening of expression libraries against human- and dog-infected sera [19] or by reverse vaccinology [20, 21]; and their efficacy has been thoroughly evaluated in preclinical and clinical trials. However, to date, there is no effective vaccine against the different clinical forms of human leishmaniases, despite the progress of the vaccines against CVL. The development of vaccines against the various species of pathogenic *Leishmania* to humans has been hampered, in part, by the inefficient stimulation of the protective cellular immunity promoted by the administration of purified or recombinant antigens. The third generation of leishmaniases vaccines is based on coding DNA, including recombinant microorganisms used as gene expression vectors [22].

Among the possible vaccine vectors, the most promising are those based on recombinant viruses, capable of expressing heterologous proteins directly within the cells of the host organism, likewise in natural infection. Vaccines based on viral vectors represent a highly versatile platform for the development of vaccines. Viral genomes can be manipulated to express any target antigen and consistently carry relatively large transgene insertions [23]. Moreover, among the advantages of using recombinant viruses as vaccine vectors is the fact that viruses have evolved as the most efficient organisms in infecting cells. After 10 minutes of infection, more than 95% of certain viruses can be found inside host cells. Another advantage is that viral proteins can play as powerful adjuvants. Besides, viruses can infect antigen-presenting cells (APC), avoiding cross-presentation. Lastly, some recombinant viruses can be lyophilized and stored without the need for special refrigeration equipment [22]. Considering the recombinant viruses most commonly used as vaccine vectors, there are already established high-throughput and large-scale production processes, aiming to use this technology in the context of pandemics [23]. Vaccinia virus is one of the most attractive and efficient vectors [22] and widely used in leishmaniases vaccine trials, which is the focus of the present study.

2. Immunology of leishmaniases

Resistance to infection by *Leishmania* spp. is mediated by both innate (macrophages, neutrophils) and adaptive (T cells) immunity. Macrophages are the main cells of the mononuclear phagocytic system parasitized by *Leishmania* spp., despite the fact that neutrophils are among the first cells recruited to contain the parasite at infection site [19]. A protective immunity against all forms of leishmaniases depends on the elimination of parasites by activated macrophages. Paradoxically, *Leishmania* spp. use the phagocytic function of macrophages as a strategy of internalization and replication within phagolysosomes. In this way, macrophages play both as host cells and as effector cells that attack parasites. Internalization of *Leishmania* spp. by host cells induces the production of pro-inflammatory cytokines involved in the elimination of parasites [11]. Activation of macrophages is firstly mediated by Toll-like receptors (TLR), subtypes of pattern recognition receptors (PRR) that play as the first line of defense against parasites, activating NFκB (nuclear factor "kappa-light-chain enhancer" of activated B cells) and resulting in the production of pro-inflammatory cytokines, such as interleukin-12 (IL-12) and tumor necrosis factor (TNF). Also part of the innate immune response is the NOD-like receptors, which are cytosolic PRR essential in the detection of intracellular pathogens. Together, the signaling cascades of TRL and NOD regulate the inflammatory and apoptotic responses of infected cells [24].

Reactive oxygen, nitrogen, and nitric oxide (NO) species, induced by IL-12, are the main responsible for the macrophages leishmanicidal activity. NO is produced from the metabolism of L-arginine, in a reaction catalyzed by the inducible nitric oxide synthase (iNOS). Cytokines such as interferon gamma (IFN-γ) and TNF-α stimulate iNOS expression, while IL-4 and IL-10 inhibit its expression, turning macrophages refractory to leishmanicidal activity [23, 24].

Dendritic cells (DC) also belong to the mononuclear phagocytic system and play as a link between innate and adaptive immune responses. DC are recruited to the site of infection by cytokine/chemokine released by infected macrophages and neutrophils. The ability of DC to present antigens through MHC (major histocompatibility complex) classes I and II induces the stimulation of *Leishmania*-specific $CD8^+$ and $CD4^+$ T cells, respectively, which are essential in acquiring *Leishmania* spp. resistance [19].

CD4⁺ T cells play a crucial role in the protective immunity against *Leishmania* spp. due to the production of various cytokines associated with parasite resistance, such as IFN-γ and TNF-α [25]. The use of murine models in leishmaniases preclinical vaccine trials allowed the identification of two subtypes of CD4⁺ T cells, which produce and secrete cytokines capable of inducing different effector functions. The studies that used as basis the model of *L. major* infection, established in BALB/c mice and proposed by Sacks *et al.* [26], defined the Th1/Th2 paradigm of resistance/susceptibility to infection and the role of cytokines such as IL-12 and IL-4 in the development of Th1 and Th2 cells subtypes, respectively [25, 27]. Generally, CL-causing *Leishmania* species require a Th1-type immune response pattern for cure in murine models [28]. Protective immunity in visceral infection is also related to the Th1 response pattern and occurs in the presence of macrophage-activating cytokines, such as IL-12 and IFN-γ, and by the formation of hepatic granulomas, structures capable of containing infection through the action of the mononuclear phagocytic system cells, which are activated by IFN-γ [29]. However, unlike the disease caused by *L. major*, the dichotomy of the Th1/Th2 immune response profile is not evident in VL murine models [30]. The susceptibility phenotype in VL murine seems to be more related to the inability to develop an effective Th1 response than in the elaboration of an exacerbated Th2 response [31]. The mechanisms involved in the differentiation of naïve CD4⁺ T cells in the Th1 and Th2 phenotypes are not yet well known, and several factors influence the resistance or susceptibility to leishmaniases, including host genetic variations, genetic variations between species and parasite strains, as well as the size of inoculum, and number of *Leishmania* spp. infective forms received by the host through the phlebotomine bite [24].

Although *Leishmania* spp. reside within phagolysosomes of mononuclear phagocyte system cells, mainly macrophages, their antigens can be presented via MHC class I to CD8⁺ T cells by cross-presentation [32]. The production of cytokines and the cytotoxic activity of CD8⁺ T cells contribute to the completion of *Leishmania* spp. infection. It was initially believed that CD8⁺ T cells performed effector function only during reinfection by parasites. However, studies have shown that they are also crucial in controlling primary infection by inducing the Th1 profile of immune response through the production of IFN-γ [11]. In addition to the production of cytokines, CD8⁺ T cells also participate in the control of infection through cytotoxic mechanisms, such as the production of granzyme and perforin [8, 33].

The wide variety of cytokines and effector mechanisms involved in the immune responses induced by various species of *Leishmania* clarifies the complexity of leishmaniases. However, murine models of *Leishmania* spp. are able to mimic several aspects of human disease, being the main source of knowledge about the immunology of leishmaniases and the tool most used in the evaluation of efficacy in preclinical vaccine trials [11].

3. Activation mechanisms of the immune response by recombinant viruses

The mammalian immune system has evolved to the efficient recognition of intruder viruses, being able to activate potent innate and adaptive immune responses (see **Figure 1**). Depending on the nature and replication strategy of the viral genome, several PRR are involved in the innate immune response to the recombinant virus (see **Figure 1**). Receptors for nucleic acids include TLR3, TLR7, TLR8, and TLR9 in the endosome, as well as cytosolic RNA/DNA sensors such as RIG-I (retinoic acid inducible gene I), MDA5 (melanoma differentiation-associated gene 5), and cGAS (cyclic GMP-AMP synthase). After binding to the viral genome, these receptors signal via the NFκB and MAPK (mitogen-activated protein kinase) pathways, resulting in the induction of pro-inflammatory cytokines and chemokines. Viral vectors that induce inflammation generally play as "self-adjuvanted." A second effect of endosomal TLR signaling is the activation of interferon regulatory factor (IRF) 3 and IRF7, transcription factors necessary for the expression of the type I interferon (IFN-I) genes: IFN-α and IFN-β [34]. IFN-I induces the maturation of APC (see **Figure 2**), especially DC, by stimulating the expression of co-stimulatory molecules such as CD80, CD86, and CD40, which in turn, lead to an efficient DC homing to secondary lymphoid organs and the antigens presentation to $CD4^+$ and $CD8^+$ T cells. IFN-I also promotes the cross-presentation of viral antigens processed on the DC endosomes to $CD8^+$ T cells [35].

While first-generation (killed or attenuated parasites) or second-generation (purified or recombinant proteins) vaccines are capable of inducing an intense humoral immune response, they are inefficient in activating cellular immune response based on cytotoxic $CD8^+$ T cells (CTL). Recombinant viral vectors, however, have the specificity of inducing an intense expression of heterologous proteins, encoded in the transgene, inside infected cells [22]. Activation of CTL requires the expression of the pathogen proteins in the cytosol APC, as well as the binding of the antigen to the MHC class I molecules [36]. The immune response based on $CD8^+$ T cells is initiated by the generation of peptides from their protein precursors cleaved in the cellular proteasome. After cleavage, the resulting peptides are complexed to TAP (transporter associated with antigen processing) and transported from the cytosol

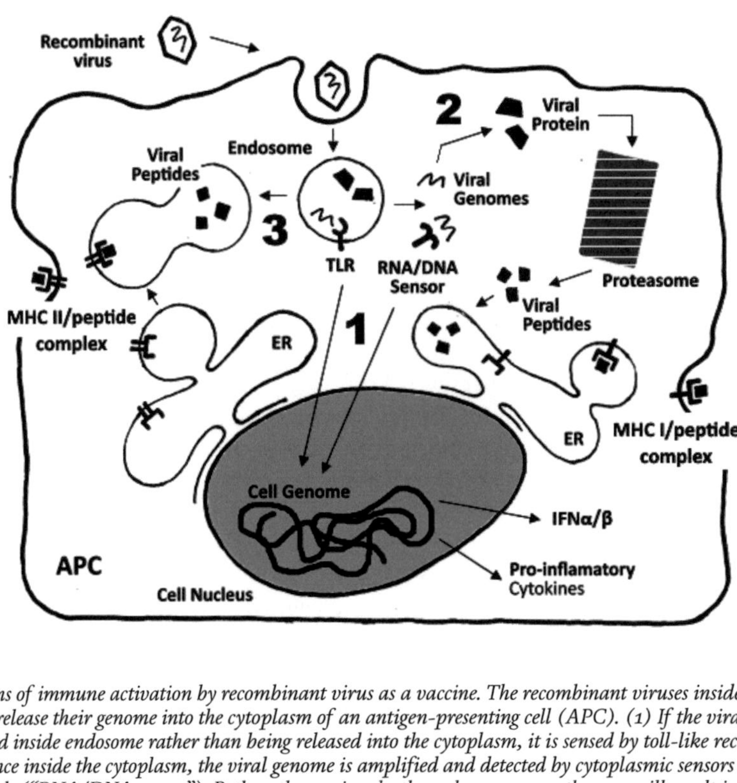

Figure 1.
*Mechanisms of immune activation by recombinant virus as a vaccine. The recombinant viruses inside the endosome release their genome into the cytoplasm of an antigen-presenting cell (APC). (1) If the viral genome gets exposed inside endosome rather than being released into the cytoplasm, it is sensed by toll-like receptors (TLR). Once inside the cytoplasm, the viral genome is amplified and detected by cytoplasmic sensors of viral nucleic acids ("RNA/DNA sensor"). Both pathway signals, through common pathways, will result in the transcriptional activation of pro-inflammatory cytokines but also in type I interferon (IFN-α/β) production. (2) Simultaneously, the viral genomic will be expressed, leading to synthesis of viral proteins. Cytosolic proteins are proteolytically digested and delivered to nascent major histocompatibility complex (MHC) class I chains in the endoplasmic reticulum (ER). (3) The recombinant viruses inside the endosome are degraded to yield peptide fragments that can associate with MHC class II molecules. *This image has not been previously published.*

into the endoplasmic reticulum (ER), where the interaction between the peptide and the MHC class I molecule occurs (see **Figure 1**). Subsequently, the peptide/MHC I complex is transported to the cell surface, and the epitope can be presented and recognized by CD8$^+$ T cells [34]. CD8$^+$ T cells recognize the antigenic peptides of endocytosed microorganisms, producing cytokines such as IFN-γ, which activate infected phagocytes to extinguish microorganisms (cytotoxic mechanism) and stimulate inflammation (see **Figure 2**).

In addition to the CD8$^+$ T cell epitopes, other important epitopes are those responsible for the induction of immune response by CD4$^+$ T cells. Viral proteins ("self-adjuvanted") or heterologous antigens fused to the viral capsid structural proteins may activate immune responses based on CD4$^+$ T cells. Viral protein or heterologous proteins fused to the virus are processed inside endosomal/lysosomal vesicles, and the resulting peptides bind to MHC class II molecules (see **Figure 1**). The peptide/MHC II complex is presented on the surface of APC to CD4$^+$ T cells. Vaccine viral vectors composed of these epitopes may induce memory CD4$^+$ T cells potentially capable of being activated by the body's natural exposure to the pathogen [22]. The differentiation of CD4$^+$ T cells in the Th1 subtype occurs in response to microorganisms, including viruses, which infect or activate APC. Activated Th1 cells secrete IFN-γ, among other cytokines. IFN-γ acts in the APC to stimulate the destruction of microorganisms (see **Figure 2**). If the heterologous proteins expressed by the recombinant viral vectors present associated signal-peptide (SP), they have the potential capacity to be surface and/or secreted proteins. When the destination of these proteins is the mitochondria or the secretory pathway, their displacement usually requires the presence of N-terminal sequences capable of being recognized by the cellular transport machinery. SP are responsible for targeting the proteins to the ER and, later, to the cell secretory pathway. Thus, these proteins may be anchored to the cytoplasmic membrane or secreted [37] and recognized by B cells, activating the production of specific antibodies (see **Figure 2**).

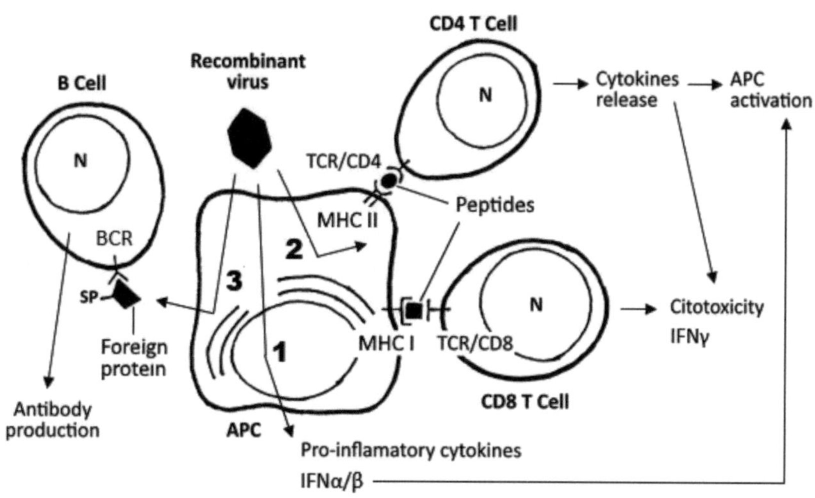

Figure 2.
*Effector functions of innate and adaptive immune cells responses induced by recombinant virus infection. (1) The viral genome stimulates endosomal TLR or RNA/DNA cytosolic sensors, triggering signaling cascades that lead to the production of pro-inflammatory cytokines, IFN-I, and APC activation. (2) Heterologous proteins are available for antigen-processing pathways, and the resulting peptides are bound to the MHC class I or II molecules, favoring the presentation of the antigens to CD8$^+$ or CD4$^+$ T cells, respectively. (3) If the heterologous proteins present associated signal-peptide (SP), they can be led to the cellular secretory pathway and activate B cells. APC, antigen-presenting cell; BCR, B cell receptor; MHC, major histocompatibility complex; N, cell nucleus; TCR, T cell receptor; TLR, toll-like receptors. *This image has been previously published.*

4. Leishmaniases experimental vaccines based on vaccinia virus-derived vectors

Although almost every viral genome can be manipulated in order to acquire heterologous protein expression capacity in host cells, not all viruses are as effective in doing so. Some types have been shown to be more efficient than others in the induction of cellular immune response, with vaccinia virus being one of the most attractive and efficient vector [22] and widely used in leishmaniases vaccine trials.

The vaccine virus (VACV or VV) is a member of the family *Poxviridae*, genus Orthopoxvirus, able to replicate in cells of several species of vertebrates, both *in vitro* and *in vivo*. The virus is the etiologic agent of smallpox. However, VACV does not have a natural reservoir nowadays and is considered, almost exclusively, a laboratory virus [22]. The vaccinia virus has an approximate size of 200 nm in diameter and 300 nm in length, and its genome consists of a segmented linear double-stranded DNA (dsDNA) of 130–300 kb. Highly attenuated strains, such as modified vaccinia virus Ankara (MVA) or NYVAC, are able to accommodate large segments of exogenous DNA (>20–25 kb) in their genome, constituting excellent expression vectors. Among the main characteristics that make them excellent vaccine vectors are (I) thermostability, low cost, and easy manufacture/administration; (II) gene expression in the cytoplasm of cells; (III) ability to induce humoral and cellular immune responses to heterologous antigens and may exhibit long-term immunity after a single inoculation; (IV) and its genome flexibility, which allows loss or deletion of much of the DNA for transgene insertion without, however, losing infectivity. In addition, in the global population, the prevalence of vector immunity is low due to the discontinuation of smallpox vaccination in the 1970s after its eradication [38].

4.1 Construction of a recombinant vaccinia virus by homologous recombination

The construction of recombinant viral vectors requires adaptation of the gene of interest for expression in host cells. In many cases, this requires intracellular recombination steps for the incorporation of the gene of interest into the viral genome. The construction of a recombinant vaccinia virus is based on a helper virus-dependent system [22]. Expression of the gene of interest may occur if the gene, under the control of a vaccinia virus promoter, is cloned into a plasmid (shuttle vector). The plasmid is transfected into a permissive cell highly infected with wild-type vaccinia virus. The gene of interest is incorporated into the wild-type vaccinia virus through homologous recombination between the viral genome and the shuttle vector (see **Figure 3**) [39].

4.2 Vaccinia virus in leishmaniases vaccines development

The development of vaccines against smallpox, which culminated in its eradication in the 1970s, resulted in a number of strains of vaccinia virus [40]. The first generation of vaccines against cancer, HIV/AIDS, and other infectious diseases was based on replication-competent strains of VACV, such as WR (Western Reserve strain), Wyeth, and Copenhagen. However, for safety reasons, most of the vectors currently used in vaccine trials are VACV non-replicative strains, such as MVA and NYVAC. Although highly attenuated vectors are capable of inducing protective immunity against various pathogens, their limitation in replicative capacity reduces their potential as compared to replicative vectors. In order to achieve a balance between safety and replication, several VACV strains with intermediate phenotype have been developed [41].

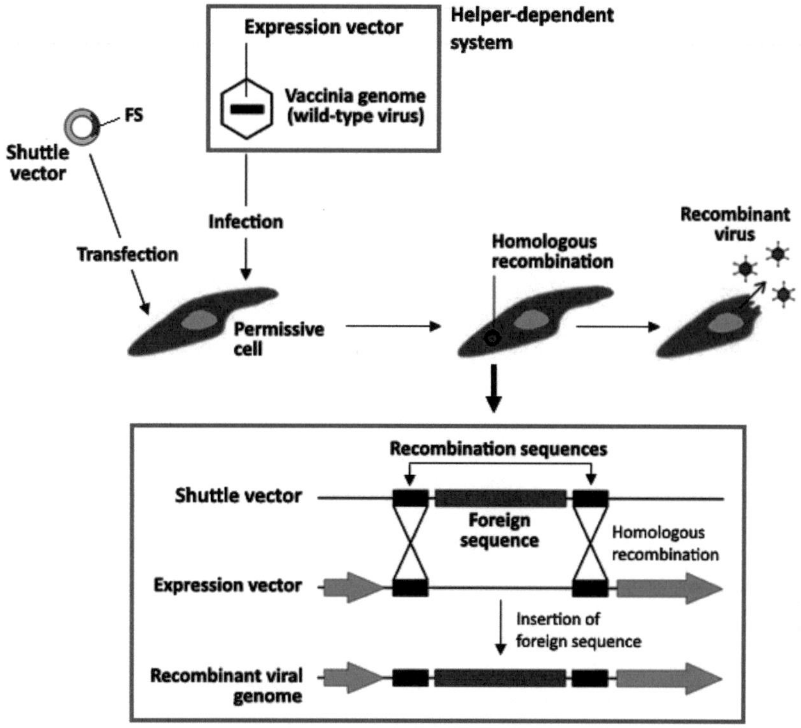

Figure 3.
*The construction of recombinant vaccinia virus occurs by intracellular homologous recombination between the shuttle vector, which contains the foreign sequence (FS), and the viral genome. Generation of recombinant vaccinia virus requires a helper virus-dependent system. *This image has not been previously published.*

The first report of the use of recombinant vaccinia virus in the induction of protection against *Leishmania* infection was made by McMahon-Pratt *et al.* (1993). The *L. amazonensis* GP46/M2 membrane glycoprotein was cloned into a live, highly attenuated strain of vaccinia virus (MuLEISH vaccine). Immunization by MuLEISH was able to induce protection in 45–75% of BALB/c mice challenged by *L. amazonensis*, in addition to generating memory T cells. This study demonstrated that recombinant vaccinia virus has great potential in the development of a safe and effective leishmaniases vaccine [41].

Since then, several *Leishmania* spp. antigenic subunits were cloned into recombinant VACV and used in leishmaniases preclinical and clinical vaccine trials. Over the past 10 years, studies using recombinant VACV in prophylactic immunizations have emphasized three antigenic subunits of *Leishmania* spp.: TRYP, LACK, and KMP-11 (see **Table 1**). Tryparedoxin peroxidase (TRYP, also known as TSA) was isolated from *L. major*, is highly conserved among *Leishmania* species, presents high expression in promastigote and amastigote forms, and plays a protective role against oxidative stress to the parasite [42]. LACK (also known as p36), the *Leishmania* homolog for receptors of activated C kinase, is an intracellular protein expressed in promastigote and amastigote forms, highly conserved among *Leishmania* species and highly immunogenic [43]. Kinetoplastid membrane protein-11 (KMP-11) is a protein present in all kinetoplastid protozoa and considered a potential candidate for leishmaniases vaccine [44].

The recombinant MVA vaccine vector expressing TRYP was used in a phase I clinical trial in dogs, the main VL domestic reservoirs caused by *L. infantum*, and has been shown to be safe and immunogenic. Uninfected, unexposed outbred endemic dogs immunized with TRYP-DNA plasmid prime and MVA-TRYP boost produced a

Antigen	Antigen delivery	Adjuvant	Animal model	Challenge	Outcome of vaccination	Reference
LACK	rVV, MVA and DNA plasmid	—	Dogs	*L. infantum*	**Prime DNA + Boost rVV:** ↓ Ab; ↑ T cell activation; ↑ Th1 cytokines; ↓ clinical symptoms; protection. **Prime DNA + Boost MVA:** ↓ Ab; ↑↑ T cell activation; ↑ Th1 cytokines; ↓↓ clinical symptoms; protection.	[47]
TRYP	MVA and DNA plasmid	—	Dogs Phase I trial	—	**Prime DNA + Boost MVA:** ↑ IFN-γ+ Th1 cells; TRYP-specific memory cells; ↑ IgG2; ↓ IgG1; safety	[45]
TRYP	MVA and DNA plasmid	Pam3CSK4 during DNA priming	BALB/c mice	*L. panamensis*	**Prime DNA + Boost MVA:** ↑ IFN-γ+CD4+ and CD8+ T cells; ↑ CD4+ and CD8+ memory cells; ↓ IL-10; ↓ IL-13; ↓ parasitism; protection	[46]
LACK	MVA and DNA plasmid	—	BALB/c mice	*L. major*	**Prime DNA + Boost MVA:** ↑ LACK-specific CD4+ and CD8+ T cells; ↑ LACK-specific CD4+ and CD8+ T effector memory cells; protection	[49]
LACK	M65, M101 and DNA plasmid	—	BALB/c mice	*L. major*	**Prime DNA + Boost M65:** ↑ LACK-specific CD4+ T memory cells; protecion. **Prime DNA + Boost M101:** ↑ LACK-specific CD8+ T memory cells; protection	[50]
				L. amazonesis	**Prime DNA + Boost M65:** ↑ LACK-specific CD4+ T memory cells; no protecion. **Prime DNA + Boost M101:** ↑ LACK-specific CD8+ T memory cells; no protection	
KMP-11	rVV and DNA plasmid	—	BALB/c mice	*L. donovani* SB-S or SB-R	**Prime DNA + Boost rVV:** ↑ IgG2a; ↑ TNF-α; ↑ IFN-γ; ↑ CD8+ T cells; ↑ cytolytic activity; ↓ (90%) splenic and hepatic parasite load; protection	[53]
LACK	NYVAC-C7L and DNA plasmid	—	BALB/c mice	*L. major*	**Prime DNA + Boost NYVAC-C7L:** ↑ CD4+ and CD8+ primary adaptive and memory T cells; ↑ IFN-γ; ↑ TNF-α; ↑ IL-2; ↓ lesion size; protection	[52]
LACK	MVA, M65 and DNA plasmid	—	Golden hamsters	*L. infantum*	**Prime DNA + Boost MVA or M65:** ↑ LACK-specific IgG; ↓ tissue damage and inflammation; ↓ splenic and hepatic parasite load; protection	[51]

↑: high level; ↑↑: remarkably high level; ↓: low level; ↓↓: remarkably low level; Ab: antibodies; KMP-11: kinetoplastid membrane protein-11; LACK: *Leishmania* activated C-kinase; M65 and M101: vaccinia virus mutants; MVA: modified vaccinia virus Ankara; NYVAC-C7L: replication-competent NYVAC that expresses C7L (gene C7L that allows the virus to replicate in human cells); Pam3CSK4: TLR1/2 agonist; rVV: recombinant vaccinia virus derived from the wild-type Western Reserve (WR) strain; SB-R: *Leishmania* pentavalent antimony resistant; SB-S: *Leishmania* pentavalent antimony sensitive; TRYP: tryparedoxin peroxidase (or TSA).

Table 1.
Recombinant vaccinia viruses used as experimental leishmaniases vaccines within the last 10 years.

type 1-dominated pro-inflammatory cellular immune response which is necessary for protection against *Leishmania* challenge and an immune memory that persists for at least 4 months postvaccination in the absence of restimulation or infection [45]. Mice also immunized by DNA/MVA prime/boost vaccines expressing TRYP were protected against challenge by *L. panamensis*. This protection was achieved specifically through the expansion of antigen-specific effector $CD8^+$ T cells. However, protection was dependent on modulating the innate immune response using the TLR1/2 agonist Pam3CSK4 during DNA priming. Heterologous prime-boost vaccination using only DNA fails to protect [46].

Ramos *et al.* [47] constructed two poxviral vectors: (I) a vaccinia virus derived from the wild-type WR strain (rVV), replicative and (II) an MVA, both expressing LACK. These vectors were used in a clinical vaccine trial to evaluate efficacy and immune response against CVL. This study showed that dog vaccination priming with DNA-LACK followed by a booster with MVA-LACK or rVV-LACK triggered a Th1 type of immune response, leading to protection against challenge by *L. infantum.* In addition, MVA-LACK in the booster demonstrated an advantage when compared to replication-competent rVV-LACK as a vaccine vector against CVL [47]. DNA-LACK/MVA-LACK prime/boost vaccines were also able to protect mice later challenged by *L. major* [48]. In both cases, protection was mediated by a Th1-like immune response against LACK antigen. However, a deep study of the immune populations involved in protection was still needed. Sánchez-Sampedro *et al.* [49] performed an in-depth analysis of the T cell populations induced in BALB/c mice during the DNA-LACK/MVA-LACK vaccination protocol, as well as after challenge with *L. major* parasites. In the adaptive response, there is a polyfunctional $CD4^+$ and $CD8^+$ T cell activation against LACK antigen. At the memory phase, the heterologous vaccination induces high-quality LACK-specific long-term $CD4^+$ and $CD8^+$ effector memory cells. After parasite challenge, there is a moderate boosting of LACK-specific $CD4^+$ and $CD8^+$ T cells. The immune parameters induced against LACK and triggered by the combined vaccination DNA/MVA protocol could be relevant in protection against leishmaniases [49].

In 2013, Sánchez-Sampedro *et al.* constructed two vaccinia virus mutants, M65 and M101. These replication-competent mutants were generated after 65 and 101 serial passages of persistently infected Friend erythroleukemia (FEL) cells. Mice immunized in a DNA prime/M65 or M101 boost regimen with viral vectors expressing the LACK showed protection or a delay in the onset of CL. In immunized mice, DNA-LACK/M65-LACK protocol preferentially induced $CD4^+$ T cell, whereas DNA-LACK/M101-LACK preferentially induced $CD8^+$ T cell responses. Although both mutants were able to induce protection in mice challenged by *L. major*, they did not induce protection against *L. amazonensis* infection. Protection was similar to that triggered by MVA-LACK [50]. Nevertheless, the protocol of DNA-LACK prime/MVA-LACK or M65-LACK virus boost vaccination significantly reduced the parasite load in the liver and bone marrow of hamsters challenged by *L. infantum*, with no differences recorded between the use of MVA or M65 virus vector options [51].

In addition to MVA, NYVAC is one of the most studied attenuated strains of vaccinia virus. NYVAC was derived from a plaque-cloned isolate of Copenhagen smallpox vaccine strain by selective deletion of 18 open reading frames (ORF) involved in virulence, pathogenicity, and host range regulation. Sánchez-Sampedro *et al.* [52] constructed a NYVAC capable of expressing LACK with insertion of the viral host range gene C7L that allows the virus to replicate in human cells. DNA-LACK-prime/NYVAC-LACK-C7L boost protocols were able to induce preferentially LACK-specific $CD8^+$ T cell responses, with a reduced $CD4^+$ T cell response and reduction in lesion size in mice immunized and challenged by *L. major*. The type and potency of the immune response induced by NYVAC-LACK were improved by C7L insertion [52].

Finally, a heterologous prime-boost immunization strategy using KMP-11-DNA priming followed by boosting recombinant vaccinia virus (rVV) expressing the same antigen was able to induce protective immunity in both hamsters and in mice against VL caused by both antimony resistant (Sb-R) and sensitive (Sb-S) *L. donovani*. Parasite load is kept significantly low in the vaccinated groups even after 60 days postinfection in hamsters, which are extremely susceptible to VL. Protection in mice is correlated with strong cellular and humoral immune responses. Generation of polyfunctional $CD8^+$ T cell was observed in vaccinated groups, which is one of the most important prerequisites for successful vaccination against VL [53].

5. Conclusion

The declaration of smallpox eradication by the World Health Organization, in 1980, and the discovery that genes encoding heterologous antigens could be inserted into the genome of attenuated vaccinia virus, in 1982, resulted in a burst of scientific publications highlighting the potential clinical benefits of the recombinant poxvirus vectors as vaccines against various pathogens. Among the most attractive and efficient viral vectors in inducing a cellular immune response, vaccinia virus has been the most used in leishmaniases vaccine trials, especially in combination with DNA vaccines (heterologous prime/boost protocols). However, studies showed that greatly enhanced immune responses could be obtained when two different viral vectors expressing the common antigen were used following the prime-boost immunization protocol, which may be experienced in future leishmaniases vaccine efficacy studies. Although highly attenuated vectors, especially MVA and NYVAC, are safe and capable of inducing protective immunity against infection by several *Leishmania* species, their limitation in replicative capacity reduces their potential when compared to replicative vectors. For a safety and replication balance, VACV strains with intermediate phenotypes are desirable. Accordingly, in the last 5 years, two replicating competent mutants were developed, M65 and M101, derived from WR strain, capable of inducing a protective immune response against murine infection by *L. major* (mice, M65 and M101) and *L. infantum* (hamsters, M65), as well as recombinant strain NYVAC-C7L, a highly attenuated vector but competent to replicate in human cells that was also able to potentiate the protective immune response against murine infection by *L. major*. Furthermore, TLR1/2 modulation may be useful in vaccines where $CD8^{+}$ T cell responses are critical. In conclusion, the potential of poxviral vectors as promising tools for vaccine development against leishmaniases can be explored by the development of new-generation vectors with refined specificity and improved efficacy through the use of co-stimulatory molecules, deletion of viral immunomodulatory genes still present in the poxvirus genome, enhancing both virus promoter strength and vector replication capacity, optimizing expression of foreign heterologous sequences, and the combined use of adjuvants. An optimized poxvirus vector triggering long-lasting immunity with a high protective efficacy against leishmaniases should be sought and can be feasible.

Conflicts of interest

The authors declare that there are no conflict of interests regarding the publication of this paper.

Authors' contributions

All authors have contributed equally to this work.

Funding

This work was partly supported by Conselho Nacional de Desenvolvimento Científico e Tecnológico (CNPq no. 306952/2017-3), Brazil.

DOI: http://dx.doi.org/10.5772/intechopen.85302

Author details

Dulcilene Mayrink de Oliveira[1]*, Jonatan Marques Campos[1], Soraia de Oliveira Silva[2] and Maria Norma Melo[2]

1 Núcleo de Pesquisa e Extensão (NUPE), Faculdade de Medicina de Barbacena (FAME/FUNJOB), Barbacena, MG, Brasil

2 Departamento de Parasitologia, Instituto de Ciências Biológicas (ICB), Universidade Federal de Minas Gerais (UFMG), Belo Horizonte, MG, Brasil

*Address all correspondence to: du.mayrink.oliveira@gmail.com

References

[1] Desjeux P et al. Leishmaniasis. Nature Reviews Microbiology. 2004;**2**:692-693

[2] Ready PD. Biology of phlebotomine sand flies as vectors of disease agents. Annual Review of Entomology. 2013;**58**(1):227-250

[3] World Health Organization. OMS, Leishmaniasis. WHO. 2015

[4] Lainson R, Ready PD, Shaw JJ. Leishmania in phlebotomid sandflies. VII. On the taxonomic status of Leishmania peruviana, causative agent of Peruvian 'uta', as indicated by its development in the sandfly, Lutzomyia longipalpis. Proceedings of the Royal Society B: Biological Sciences. 1979;**206**:307-318

[5] Lainson R, Shaw JJ, Silveira FT. Dermal and visceral leishmaniasis and their causative agents. Transactions of the Royal Society of Tropical Medicine and Hygiene. 1987;**81**:702-703

[6] Hotez PJ et al. The global burden of disease study 2010: Interpretation and implications for the neglected tropical diseases. PLoS Neglected Tropical Diseases. 2014;**8**:e2865

[7] Vos T et al. Global, regional, and national incidence, prevalence, and years lived with disability for 301 acute and chronic diseases and injuries in 188 countries, 1990-2013: A systematic analysis for the global burden of disease study 2013. Lancet. 2015;**386**:743-800

[8] Jain K, Jain NK. Vaccines for visceral leishmaniasis: A review. Journal of Immunological Methods. 2015;**422**:1-12

[9] Gillespie PM, Beaumier CM, Strych U, Hayward T, Hotez PJ, Bottazzi ME. Status of vaccine research and development of vaccines for leishmaniasis. Vaccine. 2016;**34**:2992-2995

[10] Reis AB, Giunchetti RC, Carrillo E, Martins-Filho OA, Moreno J. Immunity to Leishmania and the rational search for vaccines against canine leishmaniasis. Trends in Parasitology. 2010;**26**:341-349

[11] Kedzierski L. Leishmaniasis vaccine: Where are we today? Journal of Global Infectious Diseases. 2010;**2**:177-185

[12] Ghorbani M, Farhoudi R. Leishmaniasis in humans: Drug or vaccine therapy? Drug Design Development and Therapy. 2018;**12**:25-40

[13] Dantas-Torres F. Leishmune® vaccine: The newest tool for prevention and control of canine visceral leishmaniosis and its potential as a transmission-blocking vaccine. Veterinary Parasitology. 2006;**141**:1-8

[14] Zhang WW, Matlashewski G. Characterization of the A2-A2rel gene cluster in Leishmania donovani: Involvement of A2 in visceralization during infection. Molecular Microbiology. 2001;**39**:935-948

[15] Fernandes AP et al. Protective immunity against challenge with Leishmania (Leishmania) chagasi in beagle dogs vaccinated with recombinant A2 protein. Vaccine. 2008;**26**:5888-5895

[16] Moreno J, Vouldoukis I, Martin V, McGahie D, Cuisinier AM, Gueguen S. Use of a liesp/qa-21 vaccine (canileish) stimulates an appropriate th1-dominated cell-mediated immune response in dogs. PLoS Neglected Tropical Diseases. 2012;**6**:e1683

[17] Martin V, Vouldoukis I, Moreno J, McGahie D, Gueguen S, Cuisinier AM. The protective immune response produced in dogs after primary vaccination with the LiESP/QA-21

vaccine (CaniLeish®) remains effective against an experimental challenge one year later. Veterinary Research. 2014;**45**:69

[18] Fernández Cotrina J et al. A large-scale field randomized trial demonstrates safety and efficacy of the vaccine LetiFend® against canine leishmaniosis. Vaccine. 2018;**36**:1972-1982

[19] Kedzierski L, Zhu Y, Handman E. Leishmania vaccines: Progress and problems. Parasitology. 2006;**133**(Suppl):S87-S112

[20] Dikhit MR et al. The potential HLA class I-restricted epitopes derived from LeIF and TSA of Leishmania donovani evoke anti-leishmania CD8+ T lymphocyte response. Scientific Reports. 2018;**8**:14175

[21] Kashyap M, Jaiswal V, Farooq U. Prediction and analysis of promiscuous T cell-epitopes derived from the vaccine candidate antigens of Leishmania donovani binding to MHC class-II alleles using in silico approach. Infection, Genetics and Evolution. 2017;**53**:107-115

[22] Rocha CD, Caetano BC, Machado AV, Bruña-Romero O. Recombinant viruses as tools to induce protective cellular immunity against infectious diseases. International Microbiology. 2004;**7**:83-94

[23] Rauch S, Jasny E, Schmidt KE, Petsch B. New vaccine technologies to combat outbreak situations. Frontiers in Immunology. 2018;**9**:1963

[24] Srivastava S, Shankar P, Mishra J, Singh S. Possibilities and challenges for developing a successful vaccine for leishmaniasis. Parasites & Vectors. 2016;**9**:277

[25] Alexander J, Bryson K. T helper (h)1/Th2 and Leishmania: Paradox rather than paradigm. Immunology Letters. 2005;**99**:17-23

[26] Sacks DL, Noben-Trauth N. The immunology of susceptibility and resistance to Leishmania major in mice. Nature Reviews. Immunology. 2002;**2**:845-858

[27] Wilson ME, Jeronimo SMB, Pearson RD. Immunopathogenesis of infection with the visceralizing Leishmania species. Microbial Pathogenesis. 2005;**38**:147-160

[28] Murray HW et al. Interleukin-10 (IL-10) in experimental visceral leishmaniasis and IL-10 receptor blockade as immunotherapy. Infection and Immunity. 2002;**70**:6284-6293

[29] Ahmed S et al. Intradermal infection model for pathogenesis and vaccine studies of murine visceral leishmaniasis. Infection and Immunity. 2003;**71**:401-410

[30] Miralles GD, Stoeckle MY, McDermott DF, Finkelman FD, Murray HW. Th1 and Th2 cell-associated cytokines in experimental visceral Leishmaniasis. Infection and Immunity. 1994;**62**:1058-1063

[31] De Brito RCF et al. Peptide vaccines for leishmaniasis. Frontiers in Immunology. 2018;**9**:1043

[32] Jordan KA, Hunter CA. Regulation of CD8+T cell responses to infection with parasitic protozoa. Experimental Parasitology. 2010;**126**:318-325

[33] Brunet LR. Nitric oxide in parasitic infections. International Immunopharmacology. 2001;**1**:1457-1467

[34] Pinschewer DD. Virally vectored vaccine delivery: Medical needs, mechanisms, advantages and challenges. Swiss Medical Weekly. 2017;**147**:w14465

[35] Huang X, Yang Y. Innate immune recognition of viruses and viral vectors. Human Gene Therapy. 2009;**20**:293-301

[36] Bramson JL, Wan Y-H. The efficacy of genetic vaccination is dependent upon the nature of the vector system and antigen. Expert Opinion on Biological Therapy. 2002;**2**:75-85

[37] Emanuelsson O, Nielsen H, Brunak S, von Heijne G. Predicting subcellular localization of proteins based on their N-terminal amino acid sequence. Journal of Molecular Biology. 2000;**300**:1005-1016

[38] Gómez CE, Perdiguero B, García-Arriaza J, Esteban M. Clinical applications of attenuated MVA poxvirus strain. Expert Review of Vaccines. 2013;**12**:1395-1416

[39] Miner JN, Hruby DE. Vaccinia virus: A versatile tool for molecular biologists. Trends in Biotechnology. 1990;**8**:20-25

[40] Jacobs BL et al. Vaccinia virus vaccines: Past, present and future. Antiviral Research. 2009;**84**:1-13

[41] McMahon-Pratt D et al. Recombinant vaccinia viruses expressing GP46/M-2 protect against Leishmania infection. Infection and Immunity. 1993;**61**:3351-3359

[42] Webb JR et al. Human and murine immune responses to a novel Leishmania major recombinant protein encoded by members of a multicopy gene family. Infection and Immunity. 1998;**66**:3279-3289

[43] Melby PC, Yang J, Zhao W, Perez LE, Cheng J. Leishmania donovani p36(LACK) DNA vaccine is highly immunogenic but not protective against experimental visceral leishmaniasis. Infection and Immunity. 2001;**69**:4719-4725

[44] Matos DCS et al. Kinetoplastid membrane protein-11 is present in promastigotes and amastigotes of Leishmania amazonensis and its surface expression increases during metacyclogenesis. Memórias do Instituto Oswaldo Cruz. 2010;**105**:341-347

[45] Carson C et al. A prime/boost DNA/modified vaccinia virus Ankara vaccine expressing recombinant Leishmania DNA encoding TRYP is safe and immunogenic in outbred dogs, the reservoir of zoonotic visceral leishmaniasis. Vaccine. 2009;**27**:1080-1086

[46] Jayakumar A, Castilho TM, Park E, Goldsmith-Pestana K, Blackwell JM, McMahon-Pratt D. TLR1/2 activation during heterologous prime-boost vaccination (DNA-MVA) enhances CD8+ T cell responses providing protection against Leishmania (Viannia). PLoS Neglected Tropical Diseases. 2011;**5**:e1204

[47] Ramos I et al. Heterologous prime-boost vaccination with a non-replicative vaccinia recombinant vector expressing LACK confers protection against canine visceral leishmaniasis with a predominant Th1-specific immune response. Vaccine. 2008;**26**:333-344

[48] Pérez-Jiménez E, Kochan G, Gherardi MM, Esteban M. MVA-LACK as a safe and efficient vector for vaccination against leishmaniasis. Microbes and Infection. 2006;**8**:810-822

[49] Sánchez-Sampedro L, Gómez CE, Mejías-Pérez E, Sorzano CO, Esteban M. High quality long-term CD4+and CD8+effector memory populations stimulated by DNA-LACK/MVA-LACK regimen in Leishmania major BALB/C model of infection. PLoS One. 2012;**7**:e38859

[50] Sanchez-Sampedro L, Gomez CE, Mejias-Perez E, Perez-Jimenez E,

Oliveros JC, Esteban M. Attenuated and replication-competent Vaccinia virus strains M65 and M101 with distinct biology and immunogenicity as potential vaccine candidates against pathogens. Journal of Virology. 2013;**87**:6955-6974

[51] Fernández L et al. Antigenicity of leishmania-activated C-kinase antigen (LACK) in human peripheral blood mononuclear cells, and protective effect of prime-boost vaccination with pCI-neo-LACK plus attenuated LACK-expressing vaccinia viruses in hamsters. Frontiers in Immunology. 2018;**9**:843

[52] Sánchez-Sampedro L, Mejías-Pérez E, S Sorzano CÓ, Nájera JL, Esteban M. NYVAC vector modified by C7L viral gene insertion improves T cell immune responses and effectiveness against leishmaniasis. Virus Research. 2016;**220**:1-11

[53] Guha R et al. Heterologous priming-boosting with DNA and vaccinia virus expressing kinetoplastid membrane protein-11 induces potent cellular immune response and confers protection against infection with antimony resistant and sensitive strains of Leishmania (Leishmania) donovani. Vaccine. 2013;**31**:1905-1915